CARING FOR THE MENTALLY ILL IN THE COMMUNITY

Caring for the Mentally Ill in the Community

CHARLES ANTHONY BUTTERWORTH
MSc, RMN, SRN, DN (London), Teachers Cert.
(Manchester University), RNT
Principal Lecturer, Manchester Polytechnic

DAVID SKIDMORE
MSc, RMN, Teachers Cert., RCNT
Lecturer, Manchester Polytechnic

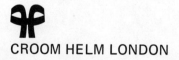

CROOM HELM LONDON

©1981 C.A. Butterworth and D. Skidmore
Croom Helm Ltd, 2-10 St John's Road, London SW11

British Library Cataloguing in Publication Data

Butterworth, Charles Anthony
    Caring for the mentally ill in the community-
    1. Mentally ill - care and treatment
    I. Title   II. Skidmore, David
    362.2'0425   RC439

    ISBN 0-7099-0071-6
    ISBN 0-7099-0072-4 (pbk)

Typeset by Jayell Typesetting · London
Printed in Great Britain by
Biddles Ltd, Guildford, Surrey

CONTENTS

Preface 9

Part One: Psychiatric Illness in the Community

1. The Road to Illness 13

2. Hospital Care versus Community Care 22

3. On Seeking Assistance and Using the Family in Treatment 33

Part Two: Treatment Practice

4. Assessment 49

5. Treatment Approaches 64

6. Programme Planning and Evaluation 99

Author Index 122

Subject Index 124

This book is dedicated with love to our wives
Jacqueline and Betty — our constant support.

PREFACE

Caring for the psychologically disordered in the community is no longer a new idea. Community care is slowly gaining a strong foothold in the principles of health care and continues to expand. Many arguments are proffered for its apparent success as a system of care delivery: for example, it is said to be cheaper than institutional care, that it reduces the need for hospital beds and negates the need for further hospital expansion. Such arguments may be minor, if indeed they are true, since the main value of community care should be that it encourages an individual approach, allows the client to become involved in his own therapy, with the view that the client takes ultimate responsibility for himself, and also allows the family to stay united.

The problem with community care is that it has developed without a philosophy of its own. Community practitioners come from diverse backgrounds based on diverse philosophies. The job of the community psychiatric nurse, for example, is a product of institutional care and consequently is already entrenched in the institutional philosophy and may be inappropriate for the community. Although the roles of community practitioners evolve via different routes their roles in the community frequently overlap; at best practitioners can only compromise regarding their attitudes towards care-giving, and at worst they become rivals pulling in different directions. To be really effective, community practitioners must develop a common philosophy divorced from their own particular disciplines — a philosophy that will unify their approaches towards care-giving and place the client first.

This book attempts to open the gates that lead onto the road where such a philosophy can be developed. It does not intend to provide that philosophy since this must arise in the field itself. Neither does it seek to set itself up as a definitive guide to clinical and practical excellence. What it does seek to do is stimulate the reader into thinking about his or her role and how that role might be improved for the client's benefit. There are guidelines offered in certain areas, such as assessment, but these should not be assumed to be absolute or complete. What we offer here is part philosophy, part discussion and part suggestion which, we hope, will help the reader to develop an approach unique to the community professional. For this reason it is not aimed at any one particular discipline; rather, it is directed towards all those who deliver care in the community — social workers, nurses, volunteers and doctors — and those interested in community care either as managers or sympathetic onlookers.

This book can be compared to a verbal map in that it seeks to guide the reader through the routes that deliver clients to the care-giver's door and makes suggestions regarding the route 'home'. We have referred to the area of medical sociology, which in recent years has done much to help professionals understand what goes on during client-professional encounters. The first two chapters explore the sociological implications of becoming a client/patient and examine the differences between hospital/institutional and community care. We have sought to make these sections readable in the hope that the reader will later refer to other works. From this foundation examination is made of the help that the family can offer and the resources available to clients. Finally the principles of treatment and assessment are explored via the use of case studies drawn from the authors' own experiences.

We have sought to produce a text that encompasses the two areas of theory and practice; whether we have succeeded is for the reader to decide. In our opinion this book would be failing in its intention if readers use it as a direct prescription for practice; we feel that no one book should exert such influence. We will have succeeded if the reader considers the suggestions contained herein, questions them and uses his or her critical judgement to develop a particular role. A philosophy can only be developed and a profession only become effective by the constant re-evaluation of the theories and methods used by those in the field. The academic world can aid in this development but should not monopolise it.

No book in the field of mental disorder can claim to have all the answers and our own biases and prejudices are only too evident. For this we make no apology; rather we would request your help in putting some of the ideas into practice in order to test their validity more fully.

The plea of this book is 'Stop and think!' Do not rush headlong into the community armed with ideas and approaches which are appropriate only to an institutional setting. Give room for manoeuvre, treat the mentally disordered as people and not as illnesses, for they are vulnerable and in their hour of need have turned to you for help.

PART ONE

PSYCHIATRIC ILLNESS IN THE COMMUNITY

1 THE ROAD TO ILLNESS

What do we mean by 'sickness'? Obviously it can have different meanings for different people: for some it may mean the actual act of vomiting; for others it means being ill; we use the word to signify boredom, 'I'm sick of this', or irritation, 'You make me sick'. However, for the purpose of this discussion the term will be used to signify the notion of being ill. It will, however, be beneficial if therapists remember that it can hold many meanings.

Sickness is something that most people suffer at one time or another. Whether their period of sickness is short or long, it creates more than a feeling of disease in the individual. Once sickness is recognised by the sufferer, it marks the transition into a new status; behaviour patterns tend to change and aspects of one role are evaded as others are adopted (Miller, 1978). This is not really a concept difficult to accept if one explores the process further.

It is during childhood that we are first exposed to the 'rituals of living' and meanings are given to 'social symbols'. Such rituals and symbols help to create the stability of life and keep that thread of normality running through everyday living (Lewis, 1976). Thus, it is during childhood that we learn how to interpret and respond to sickness cures; here too that we comprehend the positive aspects of sickness. Consider, for example, the toddler who falls; initially he may struggle back to his feet and continue his toddle, unless of course he sustains severe injury. Any tears shed at this time appear to be of frustration rather than pain. However, if adults are present the chances are that they will hurry to the infant and cuddle him, offering a great deal of attention. Toddlers quickly learn how to use sickness or injury for their own benefit and will actively seek out an adult following a fall, when attention will again be given. This type of behaviour is sometimes evident in institutions for the mentally handicapped where a child will self-inflict injury in order to gain attention. The association is soon made between sickness and attention, the latter being something most of us enjoy. Hence, attention is assimilated into the nebulous symbol of sickness. During our early development our attitude to sickness rapidly matures; we sophisticate the tool. Certain acts can be avoided when we are, or profess to be, ill. How many of us can honestly say that we *never* pretended to be ill in order to avoid school? It has been shown that children in English schools see many positive aspects in being 'sick' and missing school is one of the most prominent (Richman and Skidmore, 1980). However, to interrupt this digression, we can now add another positive facet to the sickness process: not only does it bring attention, but it also allows us to avoid the objectionable. Many children develop diverse strategies when feigning illness. They quickly learn that a mere statement of ill-health is insufficient when trying to persuade parents not to pack them off to school. Hence, the canny child allows the parent to make the suggestion by displaying sickness cues: facial expressions, lethargy, refusing a favourite meal or even sweets. Again (Richman and Skidmore found that) schoolchildren report that illness periods are parent-prompted; the parent asks the child if he or she is ill and the child affirms the notion. A little forethought and practice often perfects such skills, so that even the more cynical type of adult can be successfully duped. In another study, it was found that one child was so successful in this 'art' that he even duped his family practitioner and gained access into hospital (Skidmore and Stoker, 1974). Children are not the type of people, however, who visualise only two states of existence — sickness and health. They tend to dichotomise illness into 'rest, stay-off-school type' and 'medicine-type' (Richman and Skidmore, 1980). One assumes that the former type attracts the feigners.

During adulthood the process continues to sophisticate. We discover that it can be used as a way of saying 'no' without really saying it: 'Jesus . . . my back . . . ouch . . . better paint the ceiling another day', or even 'I have a headache', a frequent nocturnal utterance of either sex. It is during adulthood that the true value of labelling is identified. Much more can be conveyed to the potential sympathiser by conveniently dropping a choice label. Medical and anatomical phrases rate high in the sympathy league. Witness the difference in meaning between 'cold' and 'flu'. Such labels convey far more than the mere 'I'm not well'. Images can be conjured from labels: polio, for instance, may stimulate pictures of iron lungs, calipers or wasting away (Davis, 1963). Labels also suggest the type of behaviour to be expected and what the sufferer is capable of; for example, a broken leg or sprained ankle would suggest a limp, expressions of discomfort and an overt avoidance of the athletic.

Let us now consider how illness behaviour is reinforced. If one awakens one morning and does not feel too good, one might consider the possibility of illness. Initially one may try to treat the malady alone for a few days. However, should the disease fail to respond one may consult the family doctor, thinking one *might* be ill. The doctor will treat the condition and perhaps allow time off work, thus reinforcing the notion. Should he, however, refer to a specialist, it is confirmed that one *is* ill. This whole process will have been influenced by culture, education and the lay network. The actual 'patient-career' commences prior to the medical encounter, but once referred to a specialist the 'career' takes an important turn. The matter is no longer in the control of the patient. It is confirmed that he is ill, that he, alone, can do nothing and must rely on the expertise of specialists. He expects treatment to be administered, while he takes an essentially passive role. He expects allowances to be made for his behaviour, because he is ill, and such consideration will be shown by others taking over some of his responsibilities and some facets of his previous role. Thus he can concentrate on getting well again. Interwoven within the process of learning sickness-behaviour is the process of learning how to cope and respond to those who display sickness; consequently many of the patient's expectations tend to be reinforced by a 'caring' society.

Imitating sickness to punish others can be viewed as an extension of the 'playing for sympathy' pantomime and tends to be the action of choice when the display fails to gain sympathy and/or excuse from duties. It is a sort of 'You'll be sorry when I die' display much used by children and something many of us fail to grow out of. It can and does work because many people view sickness as retribution for family 'sin' (Davis, 1963; Zola, 1971).

At this stage a simplified model of the sickness-symbol can be suggested:

$$\text{Sickness} = \frac{\text{avoidance of responsibility}}{} + \text{attention} + \frac{\text{passive status}}{} = \text{code of behaviour}$$

Within the sickness-model is the labelling-model which suggests information to both professionals and their clients:

$$\text{Label} = \text{severity of sickness} + \text{treatment programme} + \text{outcome}/\text{prognosis} + \text{time-scale}$$

The above two models are not intended to be segregated and should be viewed as being tightly interwoven throughout a patient-career. One should also bear in mind that patient-careers and symbolism are very complex concepts and have been much simplified here; should the reader wish to gather further information regarding these concepts reference should be made to Davis (1963), Roth (1963) and MacLean

(1974), and on symbolism to Douglas (1973) and Lewis (1976).

Deviance

Another term that is relevant to mental illness is 'deviance'. What do we understand by this term? To all intents and purposes it is another symbolic label. We may conjure up images of bespectacled, balding men in dirty grey mackintoshes, but such imagery reveals nothing of the term's true meaning. It appears that deviance is neither defined by the individual nor by society. There are people whom society accepts as deviants because they have been informed of the abnormality of their acts by credible sources such as judges, psychiatrists, social workers, psychologists and the media. Consider, however, that many sexual practices which would have been considered deviant ten years ago are now run-of-the-mill encounters. Is this because of a greater understanding on the part of society or the more liberal attitudes of professionals? One would suggest that the latter leads to the former and vice versa, each reciprocating the other. However, let us not digress into philosophy.

The process by which one becomes deviant is by no means simple. One does not merely set out one's stall and declare deviance. In many ways one becomes a deviant in much the same way as one becomes 'sick'. The 'odd' tendencies may be present but have to be confirmed by a professional before deviant status is confirmed. To view the matter simply: an amateur deviant, by his or her inconvenient behaviour is recognised by the immediate society. At first there will be some attempt to normalise the behaviour or provide excuses for it. The normalising process may eventually break down and pressure will be put on the 'amateur', by his or her peers, to seek guidance. Prior to this stage we have a similar situation to the 'might-be-sick' routine. Attempts will be made to contain its implications in the hope that it will eventually go away. Then, by diverse routes – family practitioner, Valium, marriage guidance, etc. – the amateur deviant arrives at the specialist's door. It is here that his apprenticeship ends and his skilled status is declared. A suitable label will be conferred upon him and, hence, he can be put in contact with other deviants. Like sickness, once the skilled status is achieved a certain amount of absolution is awarded. Once the deviance is recognised by a specialist some of the behaviour is excused; the deviant no longer needs to hide it. Following this stage, and by the aid of deviant peers, the secondary normalising stage occurs.

Here it is suggested that the oddity is quite normal; many 'deviant' associations have developed because of this belief. More important, this stage may reinforce the deviant's belief that he was perfectly normal in the first place. Many professionals fail to come to terms with such a notion. It tends to be assumed that the deviant knows that he is deviant. This is a fundamental fault in people; we tend to project our own values and judgements onto others and they are expected to live by our rules. The 'when in Rome' sentiment fails to survive in reality.

Behaviour of the individual has its roots in his own culture and much tends to be learned via the 'social learning' process. If one was born into a culture where incest was the order of the day then one would feel perfectly normal entering into an incestuous relationship. Indeed, such cultures do exist and they, perhaps, think of Western culture as deviant. Similarly, in a culture where a man shows concern and care for his wife by beating her, the chances are that the male children of that culture will beat their wives and that the wives would accept it. This would be their view of normality. Trouble arises when either the wife-abusers try to enforce their culture onto us or vice versa. Intervening agents might be seen to be acting similarly and enforcing their 'culture' on clients. The professional takes his own view of normality with him to the encounter and this can undoubtedly prejudice his view of the situation. Should the couple who accept 'beating' as normal display other problems it can be dwarfed by the professional's attitude to 'beating'; indeed, the wife may even be labelled a masochist.

Unfortunately deviant labels draw a great deal of prejudice. In other words most of us have preconceived ideas about such labels. Lippman (1922) suggests 'we define first and then see'; in other words we decide what we are about to see before we see it and then, when confronted by it, see the bits that reinforce our previous definition. Prejudice is rife in the 'caring' professions and one can argue that a diagnostic label is 'structured prejudice'. When professionals are informed that a patient is to be admitted with a certain illness, not only are they sure of what they will see, but also have ideas of symptoms, treatment and a timescale of treatment. This 'structured prejudice' has extended beyond the professional aegis to influence the attitudes of the media and the laity. Consequently, we now have labels that are more 'taboo' than sex if mentioned in public. Cancer, for example, is not a word to be bandied about in a frivolous manner; it is treated with respect and fear. Unfortunately it tends immediately to conjure up the image of death and a loss of hope. However, this may be more the result of bad publicity than of prejudice. To see prejudice at work one only needs to examine both professional and public attitudes to deviance. The adage, 'Once a "deviant" always a deviant' tends to conform to the image of a fixed belief rather than a glib saying. One must be fair to people, however, and realise that a deviant threatens their ability to make predictions. The deviant does not conform to that which one normally expects, i.e. in effect he does not behave or think as I do. Consequently one forces one's own normality upon the deviant by placing him into a framework in which one can work — we give him a label which enables us to make predictions about him. The label carries a stigma with it and it consequently seems that society conspires to make the deviant conform to our ideas of his deviance. The intervening agent should strive to see beyond that prejudice. Try and enter one's client's view of normality. Richardson, convicted as a criminal and defined by society on *its* terms as a deviant, states (1980) that his criminal activities were the *normal* result of *his* sub-culture: 'Referral to outside agencies such as the police and courts would have been defined as deviant'. Rosenhan (1973) reports professional prejudice and the labelling effect very succinctly and reading of his article 'On Being Sane in Insane Places' is a must for anyone who has aspirations on objective intervention.

To summarise: one should beware of reinforcing a patient-career; sickness can have nice aspects; labels are dangerous, so approach them with caution; one man's prejudice is another man's stigma; try not to adjust other people's holds on reality merely because they are out of focus to you, for you may not be looking in the right direction.

To summarise the summary: people are complex, so treat their problems with the respect they deserve.

The Road to Illness is Paved with Strange Inventions

In the discussion above, we have concerned ourselves mainly with the individual's perceptions of direct information. However, on the road to illness or deviance many indirect stimuli can connive to reinforce attitudes of severity and helplessness in a client. In order to understand such influences one needs to examine the 'medical arena'[1] in depth. What we mean by the medical arena is the 'stage' a person enters when commencing a patient-career. Essentially it consists of three areas:

(1) The lay periphery: the area of lay referral in which information can be gained via peer-groups, relatives, the media and that which is remembered from early learning.

(2) The medical periphery: the area of voluntary consultation with the family medical practitioner.
(3) The medical nucleus: the area of referral to an encounter with a specialist.

The first area has been discussed previously and so will be overlooked here, allowing us to move straight into the medical periphery.

When a person considers that he might be ill he may seek relief by consulting his family doctor. In order to do this he must enter, albeit voluntarily, the medical periphery. This need not be at all traumatic, since the family doctor is not traditionally associated with severe illness. This part of the arena is usually informal, first names may be used and the consulting room is normally situated in a familiar place — a place which may have been visited on a number of occasions. Access to this area and the doctor is relatively easy. This is a place of prescriptions, notes that excuse absence from work and where friendly advice is offered. No real threat is offered within the periphery (Skidmore, 1980) although one should remember that some people are terrified of any doctor. Here the doctor is known, predictions can be made about outcome and patients tend to recall what actually occurred during the encounter (Skidmore, 1980).

However, should the periphery be unable to resolve the problem the patient may well be referred to a specialist. The specialist, as previously suggested, informs a person that he is ill. There appears to be a symbolic quality about the specialist label; the specialist deals with, or at least is associated with, severe illness — not for him the realms of cold and flu. The specialist can 'order' people into hospital, open their bodies and make important decisions regarding their lives. The media makes much use of his role in this context.

On the path which leads to the nucleus of the arena the patient will be offered further information via the lay network regarding his condition, the specialist and the hospital or area in which the encounter is to take place. Within the nucleus other cues will be offered regarding the implications of entering the arena: ambulances, signs directing routes to places with strange names (medical photography sounds much more ominous than Kodak), strange equipment being portered from place to place and perhaps a glimpse of some poor unfortunate on his way to a guessed destination via a trolley. A walk along any general hospital corridor betrays a wealth of cues, often too obvious and commonplace for the initiated.

After entering the hospital the patient enters the waiting ritual. In an

English hospital an average waiting time can be anything up to two hours; this tends to be expected and acceptable to a waiting patient. Naturally, it gives the patient time to reflect on what is about to happen to him, unless he can really absorb himself in any of the ancient magazines available. Eventually he is summoned to the encounter, usually via a third person, such as a nurse. He enters the inner sanctum and sees a wealth of strange inventions: X-ray viewers, trolleys full of equipment and inexplicable machinery. Again, all of these things would not unduly worry the initiated who know their function. A pantomime of introduction follows to initiate the encounter which terminates with the patient often not knowing what has occurred (Balint, 1964; Bradshaw, 1978; Skidmore, 1980). This latter effect can seriously impair progress (Janis, 1971) since information regarding what is going to happen appears to be an integral part of treatment progress.

From this moment the patient is well ensnared within his patient-career. Escape from the arena is impossible until a 'cure' is confirmed via the same route; consequently the arena shadows a person wherever he goes until the 'cure'. It could be argued, then, that the procedure is highly symbolic, in this sense, and the patient's expectations are reinforced by his perceptions and the rituals that he encounters within the arena. The deviant treads a very similar path.

The intervening agent should consider just how far the patient-career has taken a client into the arena, since the arena-effect can be transferred to him and this would have implications for therapy. Once exposed to the weird equipment of the arena's nucleus, anything brought into the encounter by the therapist, such as a case, may be viewed with suspicion by the client. The therapist's position within the arena, as viewed by the client, can also influence the encounter. If the therapist is felt to be part of the arena's nucleus the specialist-effect may impair communication. The giving of truthful information can help to erode any obstructions caused by the arena-effect and this will be explored later.

To summarise: a patient-career often carries a person into the medical arena; different areas of the arena offer cues of varying severity which are reinforced by the imagery encountered. Consequently, when considering sickness one should be aware of the effects of:

(1) what sickness means, i.e. the patient-career and sick-roles;
(2) labels and their effects on expectations and prejudice;
(3) the various stages within the medical arena, where the client fits in and where the therapist comes from;

(4) normality, which can be viewed from many angles and can be considered 'deviant' in other cultures;
(5) sickness, which can contain a positive quality for some people, in that it excuses certain behaviour.

Note

1. Thanks are due to Ray Jobling of St John's College, Cambridge, for the suggestion of the title 'medical arena'.

References

Balint, M. (1964) *The Doctor, His Patient and the Illness* (Pitman Medical, Tunbridge Wells)
Bradshaw, J. (1978) *Doctors on Trial* (Wildwood Press, London)
Davis, F. (1963) *Passage through Crisis* (Bobbs-Merrill, Indianapolis)
Douglas, M. (1973) *Natural Symbols* (Pelican, Harmondsworth, Middlesex)
Janis, I. (1971) *Stress and Frustration* (Harcourt Brace, London)
Lewis, I.M. (1976) *Social Anthropology in Perspective* (Pelican, Harmondsworth, Middlesex)
Lippman, W. (1922) *Public Opinion* (Macmillan, London)
MacLean, U. (1974) *Magical Medicine* (Pelican, Harmondsworth, Middlesex)
Miller, J. (1978) *Body in Question* (Jonathan Cape, London)
Richardson, C. (1980) *Guardian*, 29 May
Richman, J. and Skidmore, D. (1980) 'Children's Views of Illness' (Unpublished Research Report)
Rosenhan, D.L. (1973) 'On Being Sane in Insane Places', *Science, 179*, 250-8
Roth, J. (1963) *Timetables* (Bobbs-Merrill, Indianapolis)
Skidmore, D. (1980) 'The Hidden Machine', Microfiche *Verus* (Bournemouth, England)
Skidmore, D. and Stoker, K.J. (1974) 'Space Age Therapy', *New Psychiatry, 1, 4*, 15-16
Zola, I. (1971) 'Medicine as an Institution of Social Control', *Soc. Review, 20*, 487-504

2 HOSPITAL CARE VERSUS COMMUNITY CARE

Traditionally, there exist two formal ways of giving care to the sick. These processes are by no means new and one needs to understand something of their history in order to gain some insight into why things happen the way they do today. These processes have briefly been alluded to in the previous chapter, but will now be discussed further.

Hospital Care

Consider first the hospital system. This is the more formal of the two methods of care-giving, having a somewhat insular structure. It can be argued that patients are often placed in a position secondary to the function of the hospital. Historically, the hospital developed altruistically, or at least because it was felt that great deeds could be done. Many of the first hospitals in the West grew from religious organisations. It could be argued that the hospital, as a machine, has since become dominated by its cogs. Certain cogs, essential to its running, may have become more important than the machine. These cogs, the doctors and other staff, developed into their own machine within the machine. In the never-ending battle for status amongst the three doctor societies (particularly in the UK), barber-surgeons, physicians and apothecaries, the hospital could provide the ultimate in symbols. Doctors quickly cast aside their silver-capped canes and grasped at consultantships. In the medical circles of the late-nineteenth century anyone who was anyone was a consultant (Ferris, 1965; Parry and Parry, 1976). The hospitals, by necessity, had to go along with the plot in order to attract medical cover. Fortunately there was a reciprocal quality about it: prestige accrued by one rubbed off onto the other. It can be argued that the medical profession was, and still is, fickle. How impressed we are by members of the profession who trained at the medical equivalents of Oxbridge and Harvard; how we fantasise about saving the day for Kildare — most Walter Mittys have a great surgeon in them. How protective we become when our pedestals are threatened. However, the end result of this mutual immodesty of doctors and hospitals was that doctors seized more power and had more say in the running of the machine. The age of the doctor arrived. Suddenly, great doctors sprang up all over the place. Reputations were made via specialisms, often growing from motivations other than altruism, and the specialisms became synonymous with the hospital, a situation still apparent today (Wightman, 1971; Camp, 1978; Pollack and Underwood, 1968; Shaw, 1946). The status-giving power of specialism opened the flood-gates, a specialism for every occasion was discovered and with specialism came equipment and specialist referral. Many authors argue that this marked the demise of humanism in medical care (Illich, 1976; Cassell, 1978).

Consider the patient's role within this era. During this stage of medical development patients had to undergo experimentation and be unpaid teaching aids in their quest for relief. The alternative in Britain was the workhouse, where treatment at best was palliative, at worst fatal. Consequently, the passivity of the patient-role came into being. Objection to treatment methods on the patient's part was dealt with quite harshly, for it was a patient's duty to co-operate and wish to get well. Coupled to this were the doctors' efforts to make their science superficially complex: if it looked complicated this would reassure the patient that he was dealing with a person of great learning (Camp, 1978). In reality this caused the patient and doctor to drift farther apart. What a dilemma the patient must have faced, on the one hand wishing relief for his illness, on the other dreading the consequences of hospital admission.

One should now be aware that the English hospital system, which managed to influence the Western medical world, is a combination of three hospital systems:

(1) The workhouse: an institution for paupers which was made deliberately uncomfortable for the inmates, the philosophy being that it should be less desirable than a working life. It was run along very rigid lines and inmates, even if unfit, were expected to work. These august buildings were not loved by the community, the members of which dreaded admission (Lee, 1962).
(2) The voluntary hospital: here could be found doctors. In return for their attentions patients had to subject themselves to experimentation in the name of science and the belief of a cure. Some contribution to the hospital of a material nature was also expected in return for care (Abel-Smith, 1964).
(3) The teaching hospital: the top brass of the hospital world, with treatment at a price, experimentation and patients as unpaid teaching aids. These institutions tended to develop from the

voluntary hospital.

Each hospital system developed in its own way until certain political and social circumstances brought about the situations we are familiar with today:

(1) The guild-nature of doctors became eroded by the standardising of medical training.
(2) The concept of preventative medicine allowed compulsory detention in isolation hospitals for infective cases of severe diseases.
(3) The standardising of nurse training allowed greater mobility of nurses, diluting the differences between hospitals.
(4) External control of hospitals, by hospital boards and the National Health Act in the UK, introduced a similarity between hospitals. The distinguishing titles were dropped; all became just 'hospitals'.

These events, however, had deeper implications than those suggested by the sum total of the above effects. The patient-attitudes towards hospitals are just as important as staff-attitudes towards patients. Although the two are related it is perhaps easier to consider them separately.

Staff

Contrary to popular belief medical staff are human and subject to human frailties, no matter how well-trained. Human-beings wallow in predictability and medicine has strived to institute predictability by the diagnostic-prognostic ritual. The patient has to some extent become the scapegoat of the ritual; if he did not respond in the required manner, then it was his fault not that of the system. Hippocrates even suggested that the value of prognosis was that a doctor could evade the blame for a client's death. The regimentation of hospital care preserved the predictability of therapy. Given the background of the medical service it is not difficult to understand why the staff expected passivity from their patients. Let us admit that there was, and is, no malice in this demand; it is felt to be in the best interests of the patient to conform to the norm. The patient was also being given special favours (treatment) and ought to show gratitude. This philosophy was inherited from the early hospitals.

Intimate groups tend to communicate in a kind of verbal shorthand.

Eventually this develops into its own language. This is undoubtably true of medicine, where in the cathedrals of medicine words over four syllables in length can be bandied about with ease. Unfortunately the effect of such a development means that non-initiates cannot understand the language which leads to the conclusion that explanations (to patients) are rather pointless. Treatment regimes are also subject to fashion, similar to hem-lines; patients will be sat up after one paper, put back to bed after a conference, up, down, up, down as fashion decrees. In fairness, often the sheer numbers of patients prevents discussion about treatment and to some extent excuses the regimentation of care. The trouble is that once established this becomes habitual.

Another point to bear in mind is that a lot of what doctors and nurses do is routine. A common failing of humans is assuming that because one is so familiar with an object everyone else is. We assume that patients realise just what is being done when we take a pulse, give an injection or take a blood pressure. It is rather like an experienced motorist failing to understand the anxiety of a learner driver.

To summarise, the present hospital system was established in the mid-twentieth century but had its roots in history. It was largely responsible for producing a breed of people that spoke in a language unintelligible to the laity, using processes that provoked fear and convinced people that scientific intervention was the only answer to illness.

Patients

The patient about to be admitted to hospital is about as prepared for the event as the 'Happy Families' player turning up for a poker game. The very fact that he is going into hospital confirms that he is ill; he is entering alien territory about which he can make no predictions; he has also had the benefit of the lay network ('Our Jim went in there just before he died') and the pleasure of historical association. By the latter we mean that several hospitals are associated with specialisms (e.g. cancer care). There are suggestions that the patient often has no real idea why he is being admitted (Ley and Spelman, 1965; Skidmore, 1980) and he probably thinks the worst (Skidmore, 1980). He is subsequently subjected to the admission routine: documented in a usually impersonal manner, allocated a bed (which often has the minimum of privacy), his clothing is removed, he dons the hospital uniform of pyjamas and he often has to take a bath, regardless of his state of cleanliness. The ward life unfolds to him: he hears grim tales from the old lags, has the 'death-beds' pointed out to him, hears about the staff's status, has meals at certain times, goes to bed at certain times, is awoken at certain times, is allowed visitors at certain times: and then an entourage of learned persons, sporting white coats, knowing looks and speaking a language unfamiliar to the laity appears around his bed. The ritual effect, the glimpses of technology and the language used conspire with his previous expectations and he becomes overawed. His only recourse is to become passive, childlike and helpless and to give himself totally into the care of the expert. This response is reinforced by the staff and if he does not conform to this norm he may be sanctioned (Stockwell, 1972). So powerful is this response that he will often comply with treatment without question. His anxiety may be so high that he does not even hear information if offered (Skidmore, 1980) and so consents to various procedures in an uninformed manner.

The patient's expectation of the role is reinforced by the system, lay networks and certainly the media. In drama, patients are usually passive, the drama revolving around the staff; in comedy their behaviour is exaggerated and they are intimidated by the staff.

The staff-role is usually modelled upon credible peers coupled with the implied information received during training. Doctors often develop an aura usually reserved for God (Illich, 1976) and Cameron (1980) suggests that we (the public) come to believe that they are God. Nurses drop into the caring, supporting role, almost mother-like, and feel confident when interacting with their charges. They are in their domain, enforcing the rules and the patient is their guest. The nurse and patient may be equal in the eyes of the doctor, but the nurse is always more equal than the patient.

Community Care

Remove a patient from the hospital and he becomes a client. Initially, by offering him treatment at home, or within his own community, there is the implication that he is not severely ill. The attitude towards community care goes much deeper than this and again has its roots in history. All readers are encouraged to examine the history of their profession because, to paraphrase Burke (1978), if you don't know the route you arrived on you can't know where you are. How things develop historically can offer insight into the workings of the present, for retrospective vision is often clearer than the close peerings of the present.

In the UK, the family practitioner evolved from the apothecary. He always carried less status than his hospital counterparts and found it difficult to develop his own 'aura'. When he wasn't engaged in the front line of health care he could be found selling hair-pins, sealing wax and other goods over the counter of the store he ran to subsidise his meagre income (Waddington, 1977). He had, then, a storekeeper's image. Often he would be partly owned by industrial insurance schemes, the early Blue Cross or BUPA. Whether paid or not he was integrated into the community and his public felt a right to consult him in any place at any time (Craddock, 1962). The present-day practitioner has inherited this image to some extent and often tends to be viewed as an intelligent family friend (Skidmore, 1980). Also, unlike the hospital, he is usually on the doorstep, situated on familiar territory. He is not associated with nasty diseases. A plethora of technology is not normally discovered lurking in his office waiting for an excuse to be used. Paramount is the notion that he is the other half of a voluntary encounter one makes when one might be ill.

The client does not need to undergo the rite of passage to a new status. He is in a sort of no-man's-land where a new status may be negotiated, but he does not need to take on the patient-role. He may indeed be sick, but that either has not been confirmed or has been eroded by discharge. At home, in his own society, he can retain some of his individuality. He does not undergo the same ritual of admission and his encounters with professionals are on a part-time basis. Added to this, consider that he is now on his own ground, in an area where he can make predictions and the professional is the intruder.

The professional may find himself placed in somewhat of a dilemma since the client may not act like a typical patient. Clients may question decisions, even refuse treatment. The hospital professional exerts a kind of sapiential law over the patient, while a client has the law on his side. Professionals, lacking the support of the back-up services they enjoy in hospital, may feel less than adequate in such encounters. Again, the client does not have to allow access to these intruders; they can only enter with his agreement; the notion of voluntary co-operation is reinforced. Of course, recourse to compulsory admission is available, but this requires co-operation from the hospital and consequently the client can easily identify the hospital as the culprit since he is removed from his home to hospital.

This, then, is what we find: depending upon the situation of care, two types of person receive treatment — patients and clients. The patient is far more predictable than the client since his role is well-formalised; the professional feels confident with patient-encounters because he holds all the aces. The client, however, when he plays on his own ground, has a few aces up his own sleeve. He may often prove to be unpredictable to the professional because there is no formal 'client-role'.

Describing expectations about patients is fairly straightforward since it is based upon how the hospital responds to the treatment fashions. The patient invariably lies back and co-operates. Expectations of the client are more difficult to draw: he does not have to allow you access, his movements are not restricted and often he has to carry on the business of living between encounters. He will be well aware that the professional is intruding on his lifestyle; people tend to be very territorial when their rights are challenged within their own homes. The implication for client-care is that the client can demand treatment on his own terms.

Some of the simple differences between patients and clients can be represented as shown in Table 2.1. The projected 'feelings' of the last column are meant to imply what can happen if situations are interpreted as threatening. The patient is subjected to so much control that his anxiety may make him retreat more into the sick-role (Janis, 1971). The client, however, having the security of familiar surroundings about him may rebel with an overt display of anger and terminate the encounter.

Table 2.1: Typical Differences Between Patients and Clients

	Territory	Situation	Lifestyle	Status	Role	Rules	Feelings
Patient	foreign	restricted	interrupted	changed	new	alien	uncertain, anxious — sick
Client	familiar	free	similar	similar	dual or same	own	if anxious — anger

These differences have been illustrated in order to indicate that a different approach is necessary when encountering clients. Exposed clients, i.e. those who have been patients, may have definite expectations of an intervening agent. They may view him as a representative of the hospital and expect intimidation. This may cause a client to be a little bristly during the first encounter and it is up to the agent to bring informality into such situations. Relationships with clients are like any other relationship, they start with a lot of fencing — the process of finding out just what sort of person each is dealing with. This is one of the major differences between encounters with clients and those with patients. Patients do not have to know what sort of people professionals are, because in hospital, relationships are secondary to treatment. The hospital directs the patient's life for 24 hours a day. Clients, however, have to volunteer their co-operation and be committed to the treatment since the therapeutic direction of their lives is only part-time, interrupted by the tasks of daily living. Consequently, in these encounters treatment is secondary to the relationship. A client cannot lie back and receive, he has to be convinced that the treatment necessitates his active participation. Conveyor-belt care cannot work in the community as it might appear to do in hospital. The approach that the agent takes to an encounter is just as crucial as effective treatment. If the agent draws expectations of an encounter from the labelling process, e.g. 'I'm going to see a schizophrenic', the encounter then has about as much chance of a positive outcome as not entering the encounter at all. A label often dictates the approach to be used, so ask yourself, for example, do you like being humoured?

One must realise that hospitals and community are two different states. The needs of the users and suppliers differ and the approaches used need to be tailored accordingly.

To summarise: health care involves three types of individuals: the professionals, the patients and the clients. Patients and clients differ in several ways and the approaches to each should differ accordingly. It may be highly improbable that the hospital system will change, but let us not transfer uncritically such a system into the community.

A Special Note on Psychiatry

Although modelled very closely on the health-care process, psychiatry tends to be much more formal. It is only quite recently that the public has realised that one can enter a psychiatric institution on a voluntary basis. Even despite this new awareness of the public the professionals have still managed to retain a high degree of formality; for example there still exists the legal right of compulsory detention, which can be applied if a patient does not co-operate. What we also find is that in this area there is only one user — a patient. We may call them clients but deep down we consider them as patients. This may be because an analogous community field did not develop alongside the hospital. The closest comparison we can perhaps make is with that of the paroled prisoner. In reality psychiatry developed in institutions, community psychiatry is relatively new and much of its philosophy is still based on institutional attitudes. Psychiatric theory gives us many labels, but all tend to lead towards one outcome. Consequently we are in danger of entering psychiatric practice with a defeatist philosophy. Members of the public are fairly wary of 'lunatics', and the media has done a great public relations job on psychiatry. Mass murderers, rapists and child molesters now come under the collective title along with depressives and phobics. To suffer a psychological disturbance is to be stigmatised and stigma is like tar, very sticky and hard to wash off. Not only does it affect an individual, but also his neighbours and his family. It influences expectations on three levels: public, professional and patient. The person suffering from a psychiatric disturbance may be treated in the community but he does not have the freedom of the client. He is restricted by stigma and he may employ the sick-role but not be seen as sick; in fact, his whole life is changed, as we have discussed previously.

However, an intervening agent should still use the client-approach for community care. The patient is on his own territory and still has to get on with the problem of living. There are, however, further considerations to be taken into account. Apart from one's concern with the patient, one also has to consider the family, the problem and society. In the hospital the focus of attention is very much upon the patient or a group of patients. Within the community one's attention needs spreading around. Again, in the hospital, by necessity, many decisions are taken on patients' behalfs; in the community the patient cannot merely start taking decisions, he often has to be taught how to. Many patients in the community have a fear of being admitted or readmitted to the hospital. This can often lead them along the path of dishonesty (Skidmore and Stoker, 1974). For this reason the relationship needs to be established on trust and mutual honesty, a point which will be discussed later. This aspect of the therapeutic relationship is often neglected in hospital because there is more than one person involved in the case. Relationships become like procedures — routine — and also the patients have support groups with whom they identify better — an 'us and them' situation (Scheff, 1968). Finally, a regime of total care is offered in hospitals, while community patients have to participate in self-care, even if only to maintain their medication.

And so, when considering psychiatry within the patient/client model, in psychiatry we tend to find only patients, but two kinds of patients again with different needs. Table 2.2 represents the differences graphically. Notice how the first few columns are identical and changes exist mainly because of organisational differences. Even so, such differences demand a change of approach. The patient in the community may adopt a passive approach and the professionals should not allow this. Patient-participation is crucial to psychiatric community care and one would not get such participation with the standard hospital approach to care.

Table 2.2: Comparison of Typical Psychiatric Patients

	Situation	Lifestyle	Status	Role	Responsibility	Care	Focus of attention
Hospital patient	restricted	changed	changed	new	little	24 hr	individual
Community patient	restricted	changed	changed	new	much	a few hours per week	a group of individuals

In conclusion, it could be argued that psychiatry should not be a branch of medicine and that its disorders are not illnesses. Let us leave these arguments to the philosophers; in reality psychiatry is associated with medicine and the intervening agent is the one who has to do the spadework, whatever the philosophy. The association of psychiatry and medicine leads to common processes, like the sick-role and the road to illness. These should always be considered during encounters with patients in the community.

References

Abel-Smith, B. (1964) *The Hospitals, 1800-1948* (Heinemann, London)
Burke, J. (1978) *Connections* (Macmillan, London)
Cameron, J. (1980) *The Pump* (Unpublished play, Broadcast Yorkshire Television, 6 February 1980)
Camp, J. (1978) *The Healer's Art* (Frederick Muller, London)
Cassell, E.J. (1978) *The Healer's Art* (Pelican, Harmondsworth, Middlesex)
Craddock, D. (1962) *A Family Doctor's Day* (H.K. Lewis, London)
Ferris, P. (1965) *The Doctors* (Gollancz, London)
Hippocrates (1978) *Hippocratic Writings*, Lloyd, G.E.R. (ed.) (Pelican, Harmondsworth, Middlesex)
Illich, I. (1976) *Limits to Medicine* (Pelican, Harmondsworth, Middlesex)

Janis, I. (1971) *Stress and Frustration* (Harcourt Brace, London)
Lee, L. (1962) *Cider with Rosie* (Penguin, Harmondsworth, Middlesex)
Ley, P. and Spelman, M.S (1965) 'Communications in an Out-patient Setting', *British Journal of Social and Clinical Psychology, 4*, 114-16
Parry, N. and Parry, J. (1976) *The Rise of the Medical Profession* (Croom Helm, London)
Pollack, K. and Underwood, E.A. (1968) *The Healers and the Doctors — Then and Now* (Nelson, Walton on Thames)
Poynter, N. (1973) *Medicine and Man* (Pelican, Harmondsworth, Middlesex)
Scheff, T.J. (ed.) (1968) *Mental Illness and Social Process* (Harper and Row, London)
Shaw, G.B. (1946) *The Doctor's Dilemma* (Penguin, Harmondsworth, Middlesex)
Skidmore, D. (1980) 'The Hidden Machine', Microfiche *Verus* (Bournemouth, England)
Skidmore, D. and Stoker, M.J. (1974) 'Concensus Group Therapy' (Unpublished research report)
Stockwell, F. (1972) *The Unpopular Patient* (Royal College of Nursing, London)
Waddington, I. (1977) 'General Practitioners and Consultants in Early Nineteenth Century England' in Woodward, J. and Richards, D. (eds.) *Health Care and Popular Medicine in Nineteenth Century England* (Croom Helm, London)
Wightman, W.P.D. (1971) *The Emergence of Scientific Medicine* (Oliver and Boyd, Edinburgh)

Further Reading

On History

Dainton, C. (1961) *England's Hospitals* (Museum Press, London)
Lloyd, G.E.R. (ed.) (1978) *Hippocratic Writings* (Pelican, Harmondsworth, Middlesex)
Tilanus, C.B. (1974) *Surgery — 150 Years Ago* (E.P. Publishing, Wakefield)

On Encounters

Craddock, D. (1962) *A Family Doctor's Day* (H.K. Lewis, London)
Davies, A. and Horrobin, G. (eds.) (1977) *Medical Encounters* (Croom Helm, London)
Dingwall, R. (1976) *Aspects of Illness* (Martin Robertson, Oxford)

On Psychiatry

Goffman, E. (1968) *Stigma* (Pelican, Harmondsworth, Middlesex)
Lader, M. (1977) *Psychiatry on Trial* (Pelican, Harmondsworth, Middlesex)

3 ON SEEKING ASSISTANCE AND USING THE FAMILY IN TREATMENT

The health care 'scene' is crowded with those who seek to help the disabled or disordered. Finding them is one thing, being able to use them is another. There are entry and exit points in the overall plan, some of which are defined by society and others which are defined by the rules and skills of the various professional and semi-professional groups. When an individual is caught up in the system, he will observe (if he is well enough) that there are interesting differences as to the criteria which the various groups will use to define 'cure' or 'resolution of problems' which determine no further action. Each helping group of lay, professional and semi-professional people has its own definition. At what point do people enlist help or have it given to them? Why is it that many caring services are remote and mysterious to the lay person?

Self care has of itself provoked a good deal of interest in the past few years. Much work has been carried out which seeks to determine why some people can cope with more stress than others and what coping skills are needed to combat the stress of everyday life (Brown and Harris, 1978; Davis, 1963; Caplan, 1964; Lindmann, 1944).

Crisis has been proposed by some as the way in which to view those times at which events become precipitant in the push towards some disorder. This area is very complex and is influenced by a host of interrelated factors. It is not the task of this book to explore these in depth but suffice to say that familial, cultural, environmental, psychological, interpersonal and biological factors all have their part to play in influencing each and every person's life-events. There comes a point in some people's lives when self care is insufficient and professional care must be called. To say that professional care is that which overtakes and supplements self care tells only half the story. As Levin *et al.* (1977) point out 'self care includes behaviours which both supplement and substitute for health care', and indeed 'It may be historically more accurate and more practical to state the proposition in reverse: that professional health care procedures include those which supplement or substitute for self care behaviour.'

There are a variety of ways to look at entry into the health-care machine. Fanshel and Bush have developed a health status index, and, using this as a tool, it is possible to make hypotheses about the levels at which outside intervention is either sought or given (see Figure 3.1).

Figure 3.1. Health Status Index

SA:	Well-being; 'positive physical, mental and social well-being' (WHO)	
SB:	Dissatisfaction; slight deviation from SA, e.g. dental caries, air pollution, minor noise irritants	Self help will be more likely
SC:	Discomfort; colds, mild headaches, itches, irritants, but continuity of daily activities maintained	
SD:	Disability, minor; this state includes emotional disturbances of all types – daily activities are continued with significant efficiency reduction	
SE:	Disability, major; severe reduction of efficiency in the performance of functions, e.g. attendance at special schools or day hospitals	Entry of help here to some degree; still evidence of autonomy in the sufferer
SF:	Disabled; unable to work or do the equivalent but able to move around the community	
SG:	Confined; not bed-ridden but likely to be institutionalised	
SH:	Confined; bed-ridden, functional state in confinement to bed	'Take over' by the helping agencies likely to be complete
SI:	Isolated; e.g. security wards – separation from friends, families and normal activities	
SJ:	Coma; self-explanatory	
SL:	Death;	

Source: Taken from Hicks, D. (1976) *Primary Health Care: A Review* (HMSO, London).

Other factors are influential in the choice between self help and seeking medical and paramedical help. Leigh and Reiser (1980) identify (using Mechanic's (1962) groupings) four dimensions of symptoms and their influence in help-seeking behaviour.

(1) the frequency of the disorder in a given community;
(2) the familiarity of the symptoms to the community members;
(3) the predictability of the prognosis;
(4) the amount of threat and loss likely to result from the illness.

Obvious examples spring to mind; hangovers due to drinking alcohol may include severe headaches, vomiting, bowel irritation and fluid imbalance. Some communities are so familiar with these signs that they become commonplace; others may not treat them so lightly. This does not allow for individual differences of personality which will of course play a large part in determining any behavioural pattern in this area. McWhinney (1972) seeks to give order to medical help-seeking behaviour and patient behaviour through the medium of doctor-patient contact. People, he argues, consult their doctor because they:

(1) have reached the limit of their tolerance;
(2) have reached a point of high anxiety over a symptom;
(3) present minor problems which are not the crux of the situation but are used to present to the doctor a more serious problem (heterothetic presentation);
(4) need the doctor for perfunctory reasons of sickness etc;
(5) need preventive therapies (e.g. vaccination, annual check-ups) although at that time they themselves are well.

Accessibility to Resources

Given that there are various levels of entry into the health care system and a complexity of socio-cultural influences at play, how do services make themselves available to the general public and what are the most convenient points of entry into the system for (a) the patient and (b) the system?

The largest proportion of health care expenditure in the Western world goes on the curative services. There is much talk of 'prevention being better than cure', with the principles of preventive psychiatry being airily proclaimed as though the move from mental 'illness' services to mental 'health' services is going to be easily accomplished by legislation (see Community Mental Health Centers Act, 1963) or for example by the disguising of mental 'illness' acts as mental health acts (see Mental Health Act, Great Britain, 1959). With an emphasis upon cure rather than prevention it is not surprising that those people with the elemental beginnings of mental disorder are usually in an acute phase of disorder before they receive the attention of the 'caring' services. It serves no harm however to look at some of the available resources and of what use these can be to those in need. Such services can be considered using a 'Caplanesque' model of primary, secondary and tertiary preventive psychiatry (Caplan, 1964) as a rough outline, but the emphasis here will not essentially be upon prevention.

Primary Care

Primary care looks to the precipitants of mental disorder and therefore endeavours to combat these precipitants by altering the mentally unhealthy lifestyles of those 'at risk'. This is a complex subject and draws in the societal safety net services which ensure adequacy of, among other things, income, shelter and food supplies. The individual may go voluntarily to seek assistance from such agents (such as charitable funds) or the agents may themselves actively pursue those in need (e.g. as probation officers do).

One way of effecting primary care is to provide the circumstances which would allow us all to lead 'normal mentally-healthy lives', a noble ideal but one almost impossible to accomplish, since both financially and morally intervention has its limitations where there is no demonstrable disorder on show.

Secondary Care

If we have knowledge of the precipitants of mental disorders it should be theoretically possible to screen out those at risk and thereby reduce the prevalence rate of disorders. Family doctors and occupational health services should be ideally situated to accomplish such tasks, but like many other services they can be illness-orientated or operating at a crisis level, so that they are forced to provide only a curative service. There is evidence to suggest that such services are changing and that routine screening is becoming part of the role of these agents.

This area can be problematic. The assumption is that as each disorder is identified, action must be taken by the services and the 'takeover' and 'patientising' of the individual may begin (alternatives to this are proposed later in this book). People identified at this stage are often coping adequately with their lifestyle, albeit with some stress or discomfort. The caring services may well tip the balance too far by unwarranted intervention or takeover at this point, when what the person may in fact need is a judicial mix of low-key health care advice or unobtrusive therapy with the focus being upon self help. In the area of secondary care the health services could and should be seeking out the at-risk groups and giving suitable support where needed, but at the same time knowing when to withdraw.

Tertiary Care

Where mental disorder is established, and the individual and/or family is involved in the often traumatic effects such situations produce, tertiary care seeks to reduce the term of the disorder and the residual effects of its impact. This is the area where all forces are marshalled to answer the call of mental illness and the machinery of health care/ illness care swings into full action. The route, outcome and points of access depend greatly upon the organisational structure of the service on offer. Historically psychiatric services have become concentrated in hospitals, often large state-run institutions from which radiate the available services of the psychiatrist, psychologist, nurse and social worker. Entry into the system often follows a prescribed route marked by legislation and allowing no room for individual variations in behaviour. The rise of the specialist clinic for 'nervous disorders' and the placing of psychiatric units in general hospitals has done little to alter this situation (see Carr, 1980). Access to the system by the public is relatively easy, but to withdraw from it is not. Psychiatric services can be very loath to shed their customers (see Butterworth, 1979) once they have established a need which can be fulfilled by caring and curing services.

Where such services have shaken off their traditional mantle and made attempts to move into the community, access points to the service will have changed and the points of entry and exit will have become more frequent and somewhat easier to negotiate. There are well-documented descriptive studies showing the changes which overtake services which move towards the community. Some of the more important of these are:

(1) The hospital becomes only one part of the overall service on offer rather than its focus (see Borus, 1976).
(2) Role change of personnel is marked. Perceptions of disorders change and the whole-person approach becomes used (see Lyall, 1974).
(3) By being available locally the service becomes more accessible to its market, e.g. through walk-in clinics and self-referral centres (see Gleisner, 1979).

By focusing upon the individual and his family the services give more realistic care programmes and allow for self help in the community. This leads to the next area to be considered in this chapter, namely the use of the family in the treatment programme, a presently neglected area which has seen only token attempts to involve consciously the family in care.

The Family

Before constructing a model using the family in treatment, one needs to recognise how important the various relationships are for the success of the family as a social unit. Behaviour within family groups tends to be reciprocal; the behaviour of a family member influences the total behaviour of the family unit directly or indirectly. Hence, if the behaviour of one of the unit's key members becomes unpredictable, the family can rapidly become socially dysfunctive.

The family is important to its members because it normally provides a secure emotional base which buffers the stresses encountered when participating in society. As an organisation it is dependent upon its members and their relationships. If these relationships are stable, then the family is secure. Relationships become stable when they are, to a large extent, predictable. By 'predictable' one means that assumptions can be made of each person's behaviour; each knows what demands can be made of other family members, which actions will bring sanctions and which actions will be rewarded by approval just as in any lasting relationship. The stable family can rely upon its members, it can be sure of each person's role and can usually be confident that certain acts will be carried out without prompting. For argument's sake, let us construct a family model: a Mr and Mrs Average plus two infant Averages. In the classical manner, this family consists of two key members: the breadwinner — Mr Average, the provider and lawmaker; his assistant (let us ignore sexism for the moment) Mrs Average, who is the carer and carries out his duties in his absence; and the lesser Averages who contribute to the normality of the family by being present. To all extent and purpose they are a stable and happy family. Mr Average gets up every morning, goes to work, gardens on Sunday (being average in his religious beliefs); Mrs Average works part-time, cooks, sews, etc; and the little Averages go to school, make lots of noise and, perhaps, keep a rabbit. Each year they 'enjoy' their package-tour holiday and return maybe with straw hats, 'pot' donkeys and myriads of snap-shots to plague the neighbours with. To summarise, their lives are ordered on a life-time continuum. The family finds security via this continuum since it dictates where any one member will be at any time and what he or she is likely to be doing, how he or she is acting and to some extent the emotional content. The family is so close that the actions its members carry out become symbolic, portraying more meaning to insiders than outsiders. In short, families seek, find and enjoy order.

Now, let us assume that Mr Average wakes up one morning and discovers that he is not alone. He is being studied by an alien presence from another world. Naturally this alien, in the best tradition, is awkward and allows no other human to see or hear him. Thus Mr Average is seen to talk to himself, not only by his family, but also by the neighbours. He is advised to take time off work and the neighbours start avoiding him. However, the family's first reaction to this 'abnormality' is to normalise it; that is family members negate its true implication and dismiss the 'affair' as over-work, or not enough sleep or the fact that the gearbox on the car needs replacing. Finally, the family realises that the father is no longer reliable. A psychiatrist is called and he feels that Mr Average could be helped by 'coming into hospital' Thus, Mr Average is packed off to hospital. What effect does this have on the family? The breadwinner has been removed, which threatens the security of the family. A certain amount of social change is necessary within the family to restore it with the stability it needs. Mrs Average, in other words, must take on the role of Mr Average. Secondly, children being notoriously cruel, the lesser Averages could well be jibed at by their school-fellows regarding father's condition. Not only would they find this upsetting, but they may also start avoiding school. However, the most important factor is that the predictability of Mr Average has been taken away by his 'mad' label. 'Mad' people are frequently represented by the media as people who act oddly, carry meat cleavers and shout in restaurants.

Let us assume that Mr Average responds to treatment and is sent home. Does rehabilitation occur? Do things return to normal because Mr Average is given back to the family? The family has undergone change to absorb his loss; can it change to absorb his return? Remember, Mr Average has become unpredictable because of his label. The family has no knowledge of how to deal with him now. Mr Average is aware of how 'mad' people are viewed by society and his family belongs to society. How does he now react towards them? Being 'humoured' is pretty hard to endure. Consider the blind man, consider how one feels inclined to talk to him through a third person. How would you feel in such a position? What effect, then, would an intervening agent have if he tried to involve the family at this stage? So much change has already taken place. True, one can provide the family with certain skills, but the relationships may have already significantly changed in a negative way. Intervention and, indeed, education is necessary at the very onset of the condition. The family needs guidance through the various stages of the crisis and the members also require knowledge so that they can understand what has happened to one of their key members and make predictions about him on his return. Unfortunately, involvement by the caring agencies is often absent in the early stages of a patient's career. This situation is not unique to psychiatry, tending to be observable in general medicine as well. This appears to reflect an assumption that an 'illness', be it physical or psychological, is an individual problem and does not concern the family.

Trying to encourage understanding when the means to understand are absent can not be really effective; and trying to provide both at the same time can present difficulty. How then should one involve the family in treatment models? Primarily, one should be aware that a client's family has more claim on him than the expert. They are the ones who have to live with him when the expert 'retires'. Thus, they should be involved at ground level. Education regarding the condition and treatment used can commence shortly after referral. The family should not be isolated from the course of events that follows diagnosis. When people are involved in decisions they tend to be more committed to their outcome (Gellerman, 1974).

The Family and Therapy

The intervening agent should be aware, when entering a family, that the client's behaviour is reciprocal with that of the other family members. For example: if a man takes second position in an argument with his wife prior to getting into work, then pity the subordinates. Because of this 'reciprocal reaction' the disorder cannot be viewed as an individual complaint. In our hypothetical case, things, or something, has happened to the family's breadwinner, they know not what, but the family has experienced and undergone great changes to maintain stability. The breadwinner has now been returned, but is cast into a role of outsider because of his unpredictability. Likewise, Joe Average, by virtue of his 'institutionalisation' has undergone change; he has learned to be helpless, accustomed to the deviant role (Goffman, 1961; Illich, 1976; Bursten and D'Espo, 1968). To some extent he learns to be passive and indecisive. He may be unaware of the changes that have taken place within his family during his absence, changes that have been necessary and gradual. However, he encounters what appears to be a sudden change: to him the family has become unpredictable. A lack of certainty concerning relationships can be very obvious for members of a previously close relationship. One appears to know instinctively when one's partner is uncomfortable in one's presence. Hence, unpredictability can become self-reinforcing since discomfort, like many other diseases, is infectious.

The rest of the family, the 'insiders', strive to maintain a status quo in order to retain the new stability they have acquired. Consequently, only partial acceptance is offered to the 'sick' member. If he tries to force, or win, more acceptance his behaviour threatens and can be mis-read as a 'relapse'.

At this stage it may be pertinent to advise readers that the above is an extremely simplified working model and may be relevant for a television serial but quite dangerous if 'real' families are viewed in this way. Families, it should be remembered, often extend beyond the nuclear model. They may have more than two children, or less, and can easily absorb other key adults such as grandparents; and of course, they can be more contracted than the average as in one-parent families. This simplified model is used merely to suggest certain points relevant to family therapy:

(1) Treat labels with the contempt they deserve. When labels are attached to any family member, changes are likely to occur. Consider the pain of advertisers now we have the 'sex discrimination' label in society.
(2) People are not singular. The 'disorder' cannot be viewed as an individual complaint, remote from the rest of the family.
(3) 'Sticky fingers require washing.' Family changes tend not to 'get better' of their own accord.
(4) Boats are rocked quite easily. Forcing the 'deviant' member back into his previous role can threaten the family's new found stability.
(5) Bliss requires slightly more than ignorance. The amount of knowledge that the family has about the 'illness' is important. Before it can cope, it needs to know what it is coping with.
(6) People like to know the destination when planning the route. Predictability is an essential ingredient in relationships, and when eroded relationships suffer.

These points need to be considered when entering a family if one intends to intervene in some way. It is also important to remember that one has to try and visualise two points of view and two sets of needs simultaneously: those of the 'deviant' and those of the rest of the family. One also needs to consider that every member of that group considers his or her view of reality as the most accurate and the most important. A proposed model for assessing needs and taking histories is suggested in a subsequent chapter.

The above argument seeks to outline why the family is a key tool in therapy, i.e. rehabilitation cannot be totally effective without the same degree of family acceptance that was present before diagnosis. One now needs to be aware of how involved one should become with a family. It is certainly possible to extend the institutional ideas into the community and these can become an insipid malignancy to those unaware of their toxicity. When using the family in therapy one has to be careful not to take that family over. Family members, as well as the client, should take full responsibility for the programme, share the decisions and evaluate progress, in much the same way that they handled ordinary life-events prior to the 'crisis'. Professionals tend to find it difficult to accept that deviants can make judgements about professional matters and, unfortunately, many clients expect and, indeed, accept this attitude. One's own attitudes are so acceptable to oneself and it often seems illogical to assume that they are not shared by others. There is a danger that professionals can too readily enforce their attitudes upon their clients. Perhaps this is one explanation of deviance. In some cultures it is quite normal to beat one's wife, or commit incest or be bisexual. Thus, when one says 'abnormal', one is meaning that which is abnormal to oneself. Consequently, when working with families, a clear insight into their concept of 'normality' is needed.

The values of the therapist can be negated somewhat if he or she takes the passenger seat or, better, the role of navigator. If the family group is allowed to take all the decisions, plot the programme and set the pace, the therapist functioning in an advisory capacity, then greater commitment towards therapy may ensue (Skidmore and Stoker, 1974). Such a role can be incorporated throughout the involvement with any family. If managed well, this type of programme will school the family in 'crisis management'.

Ideally, an introduction by the intervening agent should be made as soon as the client is referred to the psychiatric agency. The community worker should go and introduce himself to the family and explain his or her subsequent role in the case. Attempts should be made to explain what will happen to the 'sick' member and the likely prognosis. Absolute honesty is important for achieving this objective. Relationships can rapidly disintegrate at the first sign of dishonesty on the part of the therapist. Murphy's Law (that in any given situation if anything can go wrong it invariably will!) applies in professional life just as much as in ordinary life. If a question cannot be answered honestly, then admit as much; make no unreasonable promises since broken promises tend to be those which are remembered.

Hence, the objectives of the first visit are:

(1) Introduction: say who you are, what you do and what you, with the family's help, hope to achieve.
(2) Explanation: give truthful details of what has happened to the 'client' and why treatment might be useful.
(3) Information: explain probable outcomes and the problems the family is likely to meet.
(4) Intervention: give details of the role you wish to take and the part the family can play in therapy.

If the above objectives can be met, then the first visit might help to preserve the predictive element of family life.

In order to build the relationship with the family it may be useful to keep contact with it whilst the 'sick' member is hospitalised and discuss progress and answer any questions that might arise. This helps to confirm or initiate a belief in your interest. Commitment to a project can be infectious. If you, as a therapist, portray enthusiasm, the family is more likely to grow enthusiastic. However, should the therapist stay away until the client is returned, the family may gather that it holds second place in the therapist's view. Pre-discharge contact can also be useful in order to monitor any overt changes within the family and thereby predict subsequent problems that may arise. To be forewarned is to be one jump ahead.

And so to total family involvement. The 'sick' member is returned, complete with new status. Initially it may help to discuss problems envisaged on both sides. At this stage it may be required that the therapist takes a more active role than previously suggested. The group will need to be 'warmed-up' until such time as it is practised in shared decision-making. Consider, also, that both sides may feel like strangers meeting. A description of existing problems is one of the prime targets: their description, not yours. They should also discuss how strategies can be developed to cope with such problems; assurance of the therapist's availability is crucial at this stage. Credibility is once again at risk if one expects one's clients to have problems only during office hours. The family should have the assurance that expert advice can be called upon 'after hours' if necessary. This would aid their commitment to the therapeutic role. The notion of commitment to therapy is quite important; without it therapies can and do fail (Skidmore and Stoker, 1974; Bandura *et al.*, 1969).

The rationale of family involvement should lead up to its total control. If the therapist solves the family's crisis by himself then his role will become increasingly necessary in subsequent crises. One is not merely teaching the family to cope with a 'sick' member. One should be teaching it to cope with a family crisis; members should learn how to make effective decisions and devise and implement therapeutic strategies. Obviously this is necessary to develop an effective 24-hour cover, since, unfortunately, families do not cease to exist between a therapist's visits. Also, part-time therapy is a little like part-time breathing: interesting in parts but slightly dangerous. The family, as in other situations, needs to feel in control; the progress must flow, continuously, and not be dependent upon the weekly therapeutic visit. Imagine holding up the collection of groceries until the consultant grocery adviser had paid his weekly visit; family life, as we know it, would collapse. Therapy is a little like that, it cannot tread water or be forgotten because the professional is not around.

To summarise: for effective family therapy, the family needs to take responsibility, take part in all decisions, have the necessary information to continue therapeutic direction in the absence of the professional and must not learn to depend too much upon the professional.

References

Bandura, A., Blanchard, E.B. and Riller, B. (1969) 'Relative Efficacy of Desensitization and Modelling Approaches for Including Behavioural, Affective and Attitudinal Changes', *Journal of Personal and Social Psychology, 13*, 173-99

Borus, J.F. (1976) 'Neighborhood Health Centers as Providers of Primary Mental Health Care', *New England Journal of Medicine, 259, 3*, 140-5

Brown, G.W. and Harris, T. (1976) *Social Origins of Depression* (Tavistock Publications, London)

Bursten, B. and D'Espo, R. (1968) 'The Obligation to Remain Sick' in Scheff, T.J. (ed.) *Mental Illness and Social Process* (Harper and Row, London)

Butterworth, C.A. (1979) 'Assessment and Evaluation of Patients by Community Psychiatric Nurses' (Unpublished MSc thesis, University of Aston in Birmingham)

Caplan, G. (1964) *Principles of Preventive Psychiatry* (Tavistock Publications, London)

Carr, P.J. (1980) 'To Describe the Role of the Nurse Working in a District General Hospital Psychiatric Unit' (Unpublished PhD thesis, University of Manchester)

Community Mental Health Centers Act (1963) *United States House of Representatives 3688*, 88th congress, first session.

Davis, F. (1963) *Passage through Crisis* (Bobbs-Merrill, Indianapolis)

Gellerman, S. (1974) *Behavioural Science in Management* (Pelican, Harmondsworth, Middlesex)

Gleisner, J. (1979) 'An Experimental Crisis Centre' in Meacher, M. (ed.) *New Methods of Mental Health Care* (Pergamon Press, Oxford)

Goffman, E. (1961) *Asylums* (Pelican, Harmondsworth, Middlesex)

Illich, I. (1976) *Limits to Medicine* (Pelican, Harmondsworth, Middlesex)

Leigh, H. and Reiser, M.R. (1980) *The Patient* (Plenum Medical Book Company, New York and London)

Levin, L.S., Katz, A.H. and Holst, E. (1977) *Self Care, Lay Initiatives in Health* (Croom Helm, London; Prodist, New York)

Lindmann, E. (1944) 'Symptomatology and Management of Acute Grief', *American Journal of Psychiatry, 101*, 141-8

Lyall, W.A.L. (1974) 'The Partnership between Public Health and Psychiatry: Potentials and Pitfalls', *Canadian Journal of Public Health, 65* (May/June), 204-8

Mechanic, D. (1962) 'The Concept of Illness Behaviour', *Journal of Chronic Disability, 15*, 189-94

Mental Health Act (1959) Great Britain

McWhinney, I.R. (1972) 'Beyond Diagnosis', *New England Journal of Medicine, 287, 2*, 384-7

Skidmore, D. and Stoker, M.J. (1974) 'Space Age Therapy', *New Psychiatry, 1, 4*, 15-16

Further Reading

Caplan, G. (1964) *Principles of Preventive Psychiatry* (Tavistock Publications, London)

Carr, P.J., Butterworth, C.A. and Hodges, B.E. (1980) *Community Psychiatric Nursing* (Churchill Livingstone, Edinburgh)

Leigh, H. and Reisner, M.R. (1980) *The Patient* (Plenum Medical Book Company, New York and London)

Levin, L.S., Katz, A.H. and Holst, E. (1977) *Self Care, Lay Initiatives in Health* (Croom Helm, London; Prodist, New York)

PART TWO

TREATMENT PRACTICE

4 ASSESSMENT

The principles of assessment are based upon common sense, but as this is the least common of all senses what follows is an examination of the topic of assessment giving emphasis upon what it is, which ways it may lead the care-giver and finally some basic rules for the care-giver to follow.

Many health care-givers are often heard to despair of having made any progress with those they have sought to assist. Upon closer examination it becomes apparent that such despair is based upon inadequate or totally absent baseline assessments and measures of effectiveness (Butterworth, 1979). The apparent intractability of severely disturbed or hopelessly neurotic individuals and/or families is rarely as rigid as we are led to believe. Many changes do take place and numerous activities are carried out without the giver or the recipient being aware that they have occurred. This leads to the first consideration of this chapter, namely the route that should be followed by those considering an assessment and evaluation programme.

How Are We Trying to Assess?

There are two main paths to assessment and each has its advocates who are convinced that theirs is the most effective route. On the one hand are the 'incrementalists', the small-problem solvers who struggle manfully from the resolution of one small problem to a soul-searching consideration of the next. They move along an inexhaustable supply of problems and conscientiously evaluate their success (seldom failure) in each problem area. Their main criteria are high client-selectivity procedures and the total compliance of the client in whatever activities are prescribed. The scientific procedures they adopt are faultless and each programme is carefully organised along a defined route which has its starting point at a clearly stated baseline. Their incrementalist behaviour has obvious difficulties, since the complexity of man is unaccounted for, and the factors which are inextricably linked in a presenting disorder are artificially divided and picked clean of their interwoven connections which have little but nuisance value to such care-givers.

The second path is trodden by those who are basically overwhelmed by man's complexity. Such 'universalists' are presented by such an avalanche of information that they do not know where to begin and so they set out to collect all the information they can in order to find some meaning in the presented disorder. Their route to a decision is measured in years not days and demands a commitment not normally available to the average care-giver. No stone is left unturned, no chance remark ignored and every word has meaning and significance.

There are few absolute extreme practitioners. They do exist, but more common are those who lean by varying degrees one way or the other. Between thesis and antithesis there always lies synthesis and it is within this area that work usually bears most fruit for use at a clinical level, and rarely does it suffer the tortures of partisanship which occur at the ends of the scale. In this case, on the one hand it is vital to take account of man's complexity, while on the other we must give sequence and order to care delivery or it becomes meaningless.

The reader may gain further insight into two useful areas which lie closer to the midline than either of the above extremes. These two, Problem-orientated Approaches and Systems Approaches both hold key concepts which will be of use to the care-giver in the community.

Problem-orientated Approaches

The use of problem-orientated records (POR) has gained momentum since Weed (1968) and then Ryback (1977) gave form to this concept. Examples of such ideas in practice are now quite numerous (Wolley and Kane, 1977; Gahan, 1976) and a number of professional groups, most notably the nursing profession, have proposed an outline to their educational syllabuses through this medium.

The move towards problem-orientated records arose from a dissatisfaction with discipline-based data compared to a broad-content data base. Such discipline orientation has emphasis upon data collection, rather than on the transposition of data into meaningful records (thereby providing resolution of given problems). This situation has been compounded by the ever-increasing amount of information being presented by different care groups whose interests are within specific assessment areas such as psychology and social work. The refinement of their assessment techniques has progressed rapidly, but the comprehensive collection of this information into usable data for a multi-disciplinary approach to care has not. A central data collection point which is usable and easily understood by all members of a care team is essential to a comprehensive care programme.

Problem orientation provides the means towards planned care; as problems are presented then each will need resolution. To determine a route to resolution then a comprehensive means to assessment must become part of the whole programme. The system can be viewed thus:

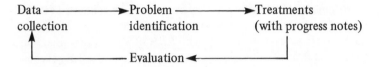

Such an approach is self-feeding and therefore sensitive to change, which is essential to a programme of care if it is to be useful. All too often prescribed routes of care are continued long after their usefulness has ceased and in some cases where such continuance is having a deleterious effect.

The major idea behind a problem-orientated approach is its multi-disciplinary involvement. It allows each professional group to have its say, make its specialist assessment and provide its data. Such an approach sees as vital the drawing together of all the information into problem identification procedures which are listed out from the presented data. When the problems have been listed then routes can be sought as to their resolution. Consequently such resolution (or at least its progression) can then be evaluated.

This system has decided advantages over the mayhem which reigns in present psychiatric practice. Each discipline needs to have its say; each needs to know the presenting problem as it and others see it; clear lines of progress can be defined and each will know what the other is doing. Conversely, there are criticisms of the problem-orientated approach. It occasionally makes little or no allowance for the patient to have a say in treatment. The emphasis is upon sorting out the work being undertaken by the various disciplines, which is fine for the care-giver but may lose sight of the patient and his family altogether. The organisational adjustment required to bring together the 'team' is enormous and it is impossible to expect a sudden rallying under the flag 'POR' of old and ill-trusted enemies each of whom is concerned for his own empire. Where it has been implemented there is evidence of a leading or dominant team member. The principles involved, however, retain their usefulness even when the system cannot be applied to the last letter.

The 'Systems' Approach

That 'man is more than the sum of his parts' is a concept which is often forgotten by many care-givers. The very nature of man's existence rests upon a vast network of social, biological and behavioural influences, all of which interact one with another to produce the end result, 'individualism'.

Within psychiatry in recent years there have been isolated attempts to apply a structured concept to this complex area through the medium of the 'systems' approach. As Lewis *et al.* (1978) point out the 'focus has moved from classification and description to individual psychodynamics — not what was wrong, but why the person behaved differently' and from such beginnings the theoretical base has widened even further. Davies (1976), quoting Mayer, says she pinpoints three topics which are central to the discussion of systems theory and social work:

(1) The identification of goals.
(2) The recognition of environmental factors.
(3) The need to learn to live with uncertainty.

Goal Identification

This subject was central to the theme of the preceding section on problem-orientated approaches and forms part of the necessary moves within systems-thinking as applied to the topic of psychiatric care in the community. Who identifies the goals and to what purpose? Should it be the professional worker defining goals for the patient or should the patient have a say; and his family; and the community? What levels of care or cure are services aiming at, what can be defined as better and what repercussions will such improvements have upon other elements in the system? Such disciplining procedures must be learned and made coherent for any service to be truly effective.

Environmental Factors

Environmental factors can seem to be very complex to any worker when they are first considered and taken account of in the assessment. Just as the patient is involved in a complexity of interlocking influences (see Figure 4.1) so is the care-giver part of his or her own life-model which is likely to be equally complex. Thus the meeting of these two will bring with it the experiences, constraints and expectations of each, which directly affect the giving of care.

Assessment

Figure 4.1: A 'Systems' View of Care-giving

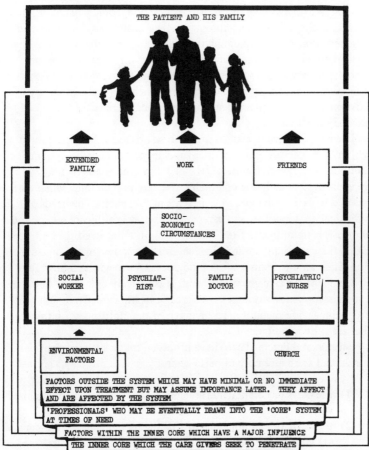

Living with Uncertainty

There is a great deal of comfort to be gained from constancy. Within rigid health care organisations there are predetermined routes along which the various 'illnesses' will move with no allowance made for individual differences. This inflexible and machine-like system is fine for the organisation but totally unsuitable for those mentally disordered it purports to help.

An institutionalised and inaccessible psychiatric service can be described in systems terminology as being 'closed'; in other words it processes, diagnoses and discharges the mentally disordered without doing anything for them other than making them fit the psychiatric 'rule book'. An example of this is the desperate urgency which is given to finding the 'correct' diagnoses to a set of symptoms. Much learned argument is given to finding the right label but once that label has been applied much of the urgent activity dissipates into making sure the illness conforms with (a) the organisation and (b) its textbook presentation. 'Closed' services give nothing away which is of value, for they exist only to satisfy themselves and their fodder consists of the mentally disordered.

The happiest circumstances in which to be caught in are found within 'dynamic systems' (another fundamental concept in systems terminology). Health care services which have the qualities of a dynamic system will have comprehensive care programmes which are tailored to each individual who presents needing help. The needs of the individual are identified and catered for by this health care service and emphasis is upon the way the system can best tailor itself to these needs rather than remoulding the individual into the 'ways' of the organisation. Such an uncertainty of method does not provide a comfortable environment for care-givers but comfort is scarcely one of the better known rewards for working in this area of health care. To mount these programmes due account must be taken of the multitude of influences that are shown in Figure 4.1.

Beishon and Peters (1976) have proposed that a system might be considered as an assembly of parts where:

(1) the parts or components are connected together in an organised way;
(2) the parts or components are affected by being in the system and are changed by leaving it;
(3) the assembly does something;
(4) the assembly has been identified by a person as being of special interest.

Such a systems model is represented in Figure 4.1. While this is by no means an exhaustive model, it does account for a number of important factors.

Assessment

What Are We Trying to Assess?

Assessment has been likened to the unravelling of a puzzle or at least the finding of the pieces (Cambrill, 1977) and as with the puzzle-solving techniques which an individual may employ, the right approach to assessment may save time, improve the clarity of the overall picture and provide a secure platform of baseline information from which to launch a care programme. Take for example the case of a man who is seen from a distance waving in your direction but it is too remote for you to discern his facial expression. What interpretation could be put upon this behaviour? Is it perhaps a friendly gesture or is he merely trying to attract your attention in order that you may help him? Without an adequate knowledge of the antecedent events and the consequences related to this behaviour you cannot give any meaningful interpretation to its display. This man may well have been struck by a flying saucer which at this very moment is about to strike you from behind, this being his very reason for waving in the first place!

This takes us to an alternative choice in assessment; should it be a topographic approach or functional in its analysis? Topographic analysis merely describes the form of a given behaviour (as in the waving man vignette); functional analysis takes account of the preceding events and the consequences relating to a given behaviour. Medical diagnosis, which is prevalent in psychiatry, serves only a topographic function and cannot give any form to assessment. A wider approach is in fact essential and it is necessary to carry this out through an assessment of verbal, behavioural, affective and social components of an individual's presentation.

If this wider approach is now employed, how is it possible to collect the information which is needed for a comprehensive assessment? Various types of assessment will now be considered.

(1) General Clinical Assessment

This is a standardised assessment for items such as activities of daily living (dressing, washing, bathing, feeding, etc.). This would seek a baseline of the performance of simple tasks through questioning an informant. This approach is based upon the informant's verbal responses and therefore there are few checks as to its validity. The questioner and the respondent are reliant upon each understanding the communication of the other and dependent upon the norms, values and culture of both parties. An illustration of measured self-performance can be taken from league football where each team considers itself fully proficient in the art until it moves up a league, and only then does it realise the limitations of its own performance when faced with new criteria. It is possible however to develop self-report measures which have validity (see Skidmore and Stoker, 1975).

(2) Functional Assessment

This type of assessment differs from the above in that it is not dependent upon a question-answer routine. Functional assessment involves observed performance of the deficits or advantages that people have. How can an example of family disharmony or social skills incompetence be better assessed than by seeing it 'in action'? By an observation of various behaviours or activities it is possible to obtain a far more accurate picture of an overall situation. This is best carried out by trained observers as there are specific criteria which must be sought out and measured.

(3) Environmental/Social Assessment

Through the means of direct observation and report from the respondent it is possible to examine such areas as (i) home facilities, (ii) activity or passivity of extended families, and (iii) support networks. These and many other factors are essential to the complete assessment picture. In addition psysiological measures may be necessary through physical examination, reports may be needed from significant others and so on.

The list appears endless but it is essential to draw a line around a given case and to include within it material germane to a comprehensive assessment. Thereafter it is possible to go off tangentially and examine in detail specific areas. For example, consider a single, middle-aged man with a geographically distant family who are seldom seen. Repeated episodes of his psychotic behaviour are now controlled with intramuscular medication and psychological support. If such a man were to present with an upsurge in odd behaviour, the following could be seen to be areas of importance for assessment:

(1) General Clinical Assessment: (a) coping capacity (current cf. usual)
                                             (b) social situation
                                             (c) financial situation
                                             (d) behaviour pattern

(2) Physiological Assessment: (a) medication (i) effectiveness
                                                                             (ii) using habits
                                                                             (iii) adverse effects

	(b) physical examination
(3) Environmental/Social Assessment:	(a) support network
	(b) precipitant problems
	(c) interpersonal skills

Having completed a broad assessment of the individual three areas, these may present themselves to the assessor for closer examination and might consequently subdivide into more detailed assessment areas.

(1) Interpersonal Skills:	(a) speaking skills
	(b) social routines
	(c) meshing skills
	(d) listening skills
(2) Medication Using Habits:	(a) consistency of dosage
	(b) use of medication for side effects
	(c) user levels of interacting agents (e.g. alcohol)
(3) Support Networks:	(a) family evaluation
	(b) support services use (professional)
	(c) support services use (voluntary)
	(d) neighbourhood antipathy/hostility/rating

Moving from the general to the particular will provide a comprehensive picture of how this individual is functioning, in what circumstances, and what resources are available for future care programmes.

The place of assessment and evaluation of mental disorder and the success of intervention by care-agents becomes imposing and complicated when first viewed by the uninitiated. Complex words, born of the jargon of health care professionals, abound, and set traps await the novitiate care-giver. If this area is so fraught with problems is it worth the effort of consideration? The answer must be an unqualified yes. Without order the delivery of care is meaningless and without checks on its effectiveness through evaluation, there is no measure of its worth.

An Approach to Assessment

Rather than taking pencil-and-paper tests to an encounter it is more desirable if a therapist develops an objective approach of on-going assessment. This need not be completed during the first encounter, but can be based over a period of time whilst the client-therapist relationship is being built up. For argument's sake let us call such an approach 'The Process of Therapeutic Detection'. Consider the following *suggested* approach, which is based upon the previous discussion. The following is not necessarily laid out in an order that should be followed, but is suggested in a form that can be developed from natural conversations with clients.

The first 'item' is based upon the notion that the reasons for your interventions are not focused on just one person. To gauge the effects of the crisis the therapist would need to know:

(1) How Many People Are Involved?

This would help to deduce the consequences of non-intervention and have implications for outcome and possible rehabilitation. It would also help the therapist to plan future help regarding family therapy and aid in the observation of sub-problems, e.g. school-phobia.

(2) What Are the Presenting Problems?

What one should be interested in here are those things that the whole family sees as problems, not your own view. You should be particularly interested in their descriptions of any behavioural excesses or deficits; e.g. excess irritability or a lack of interest. A true picture of these problems would be important when planning the future treatment programme.

(3) Are There Any Related Problems Dependent upon the Outcome of the Presenting Problem?

By this we mean that the problem which is presenting may have generalised. Consider, for example, the agoraphobic; the presenting problem may be described as a fear and avoidance of going out, but the related problems may include being unable to go shopping, to work or to socialise. The presenting problem may become lost in the quagmire of associated related problems. However, a client would not automatically start to socialise again once the presenting problem had been relieved, but certainly could not be encouraged to socialise while the presenting problem existed. This complication would apply to relationship problems within the family: a relationship may have started to break down because of the psychological disturbance of one family member. From there the relationship crisis gets carried along on its own momentum and would not be resolved by merely solving the psychological problem.

(4) Functional Analysis

(4.1) Who Primarily Defined the Problem and Was Responsible for the Client Seeking Help? This is important because it gives some idea of the family's pecking order and of who is influential as far as the client is concerned, both within and outside the family circle. It would also throw some light upon the acceptability of the client, e.g. if the referral came from outside the family it could suggest that the family finds the client's behaviour quite acceptable. These points will be useful later when planning a treatment programme.

(4.2) What Are the Possible Consequences of an Unresolved Problem? This is particularly important when one considers the growing caseloads of community workers. A therapist can only do so much; if he has too many clients on his books they all suffer from indirect neglect. Hence, this question will help the therapist assess: Is intervention necessary at all, immediately or can it wait? Do changes need to be made in the client's and/or family's behaviour, or do the members need counselling in order to come to terms with a new situation?

(4.3) What Gains and Losses Would Result from Problem Resolution? Obviously, one would assume that if a client has arrived seeking help then he and his family have been suffering and the relief of such suffering would be a positive gain. However, one should look beyond this and consider the implications of a successful resolution. Some of the family members may prefer the present situation, as discussed earlier, and resolution may cause disintegration of the family unit if steps are not taken to counteract this at the onset of therapy.

(4.4) Is the Problem Bonded to a Particular Situation or Does it Appear Idiopathic? In other words, does a certain situation precipitate an exacerbation of the problem? For example: does the husband only experience panic attacks when his wife prepares to leave for evening classes, or does it occur at any time? This, again, carries implications for the total understanding of the problem and the planning of remedial measures.

(5) Self Control

A therapist needs to know, prior to formulating treatment plans, how much the situation is, or can be, controlled by the client.

(5.1) To What Extent Does the Family Achieve Control over the Situation? If it can control the situation to some degree it implies that there is some recognition of the problem, motivation to change and acceptance of responsibility.

(5.2) Is There Evidence of Avoidance and/or Substitution Behaviour? Does the client and/or the family refuse to recognise the problem or attempt to hide and excuse it by adopting the sick-role?

(5.3) What Credibility Do Other Family Members Hold in the Client's View? There is no point in considering the use of family members in therapy if the client hates them, or feels they are useless or incompetent, and is using his problem as a means to rid himself of them. The same applies to the family's attitude – it might want him to get worse so that he can be packed off to an institution.

(5.4) Has the Family Any Mutual Strengths? There may be aspects of family life on which to build a treatment programme. For example: do family members love each other, enjoy each other's company and carry out social activities together? These 'strengths' can be used as reinforcers in a treatment programme.

(6) Social Aspects

(6.1) What Sanctions Are Being Applied to the Client by Family Members and/or Relevant Others? This could also provide information about patterns of influence, e.g. who enforces rules and has leadership influence on the client? It is also useful to reverse the direction of the question in order to discover whether or not the client himself applies sanctions to his family and friends.

(6.2) If Therapeutic Goals Are Established, Will the Family Reinforce? Remember it can be beneficial to some family members if the sick-role is maintained; it is wise to be forewarned of such attitudes.

(6.3) Are There Other Limiting Factors Involved in the Situation? For example: are the relationships of those involved in the problem so poor that it negates the possibility of resolution? The presenting problem

Assessment

may be secondary to a relationship problem or, indeed, a sexual problem.

(7) Treatment/Resolution

This part of the assessment process would strive to gather information useful when planning the actual treatment programme.

(7.1) What Does the Family Value? Once values are identified they can be used as part of the reinforcement package of treatment contracts. Such values may be social approval, relationship-security and sex.

(7.2) Is the 'Illness' a Primary or Secondary Factor? This question takes us back to the question 'Is intervention necessary?' The presenting problem could be a consequence of marital disharmony. In such a case protracted treatment would prove fruitless and referral to marriage guidance or some other agency would be more appropriate. If the problem is primary and causing relationship disturbances then intervention is justified.

(7.3) Does Any Other Agency Need to be Involved? It is impossible for one person to help everybody. Never be too proud to call in the help and advice of other experts – one cannot know everything about life. Certain problems, such as sexual dysfunction, can potentiate presenting problems. However, the intervening agent may have little experience or interest in such problems and could place the whole therapy in danger if he or she tries to go it alone.

(7.4) How Successful has the Family Been in Achieving its Goals and is the 'Problem' Recent? This would carry implications for the family's functioning as a unit and provide some idea as to its security and strength. The history of the presenting problem is important in that it can give some idea of how well entrenched the situation has become. The family may have become very adept at using avoidance behaviour.

(7.5) Is the Family Accurate and Agreed on the Problem Definition? The therapist should strive to gather a total picture which all family members can identify with. If more credence is given to one particular member it suggests that the therapist is taking sides and could result in family members opting out of therapy.

(7.6) Is Scapegoating Evident? Is one member of the family held more

responsible for the problem; i.e. the 'its-all-his-fault' effect? This would add more information to the general picture of family relationships and patterns of influence.

(7.7) To What Extent Can the Situation be Modified? This is the time for honesty. Can you really do something constructive or is the problem so vast that the best thing to do is withdraw or refer elsewhere? It may hurt to admit it, but there will be some clients for whom you can do nothing. If you persist after recognising this fact the credibility of all intervening agents will suffer in the client's point of view. In other words you could spoil the chances of another therapist who could be effective.

(7.8) Are There Any Antagonistic Responses from Any Family Members? Another cross-referral here, do all family members want the situation to change or is a member likely to prove destructive in therapy?

It is argued that such an approach, discussed above, would provide the agent with a method of gaining a clearer picture of clients' problems. To some extent it would guard against the labelling trap, but this depends very much on the attitude of the agent. It is stressed that the above approach is not a rule of thumb and agents, and their clients, should feel free to expand and modify the process.

All assessment techniques tend to be more effective when done objectively, and this is the real problem, for apart from being objective the agent has to build up a relationship. The building of a relationship is bound to lead to emotional involvement, whether this is affection or dislike, which in turn tends to erode objectivity. It is impossible to offer constructive guidance on this point, since we find ourselves in a conundrum: assessment is important for effective therapy but a good relationship is equally important, sometimes more so. If, then, the assessment becomes suspect it is suggested that the agent strives to develop a strong relationship at the expense of assessment. The initiation and maintenance of relationships will be discussed later. It is quite difficult to offer theoretical guidance regarding assessment techniques since much of it tends to be intuitive. However, on-going methods appear to work best because people tend to be more honest with each other when they know one another. Dishonest responses to assessment questions are about as useful as guesswork, informed or otherwise. The staccato process of pencil-and-paper tests also tends to be off-putting.

Consequently, it is suggested that agents develop a method that will flow and be meshed into the ordinary conversation.

References

Beishon, R.J. and Peters, G. (eds.) (1976) *Systems Behaviour* (Harper and Row for Open University Press, London)

Butterworth, C.A. (1979) 'Assessment and Evaluation of Patients by Community Psychiatric Nurses' (Unpublished MSc thesis, University of Aston in Birmingham)

Cambrill, E. (ed.) (1977) *Behaviour Modification, Handbook of Assessment, Intervention and Evaluation* (Jossey Bass, San Francisco)

Davies, M. (1976) 'Systems Theory and Social Work' in Beishon, R.J. and Peters, G. (eds.) *Systems Behaviour* (Harper and Row for Open University Press, London)

Gahan, K.A. (1976) 'Using Problem Orientated Records in Psychiatric Nursing', in Kneisl, C.R. and Wilson, H.S. (eds.) *Current Perspectives in Psychiatric Nursing* (C.V. Mosby, St Louis)

Lewis, J.M., Beavers, W.R., Gossett, J.T. and Phillips, V.A. (1978) *No Single Thread, Psychological Health in Family Systems* (Macmillan, New York)

Ryback, R.S. (1977) *The Problem Orientated Record in Psychiatry* (Grune and Stratton, New York)

Skidmore, D. and Stoker, M.J. (1975) 'Patients as Therapists', *New Psychiatry, 2*, 7, 12-13

Weed, L.L. (1968) 'Medical Records that Guide and Teach', *New England Journal of Medicine, 278*, 593-600 and 652-7

Wolley, F.R. and Kane, R.L. (1977) 'Improving Patient Care through the Interdisciplinary Record' in Reinhardt, A.M. and Quinn, M.D. (eds.) *Current Practise in Family Centered Community Nursing* (C.V. Mosby, St Louis)

Further Reading

Cambrill, E. (ed.) (1977) *Behaviour Modification, Handbook of Assessment, Intervention and Evaluation* (Jossey Bass, San Francisco)

Lewis, J.M., Beavers, W.R., Gossett, J.T. and Phillips, V.A. (1978) *No Single Thread, Psychological Health in Family Systems* (Macmillan, New York)

5 TREATMENT APPROACHES

The title of this chapter is perhaps a little misleading when applied to psychiatric intervention. It implies an illness which requires remedial action. We have previously discussed the possibility that readjustment, rather than treatment, may be appropriate in some psychological problems. However, rather than rewrite psychiatric nomenclature, it is felt to be more practical if recognised terms are used here.

Treatment can rarely be delivered in package form. In the field of psychiatry one is dealing with an individual or a group of individuals rather than a disease. It is a fact of life that people are different; this may add to the spice of life but it is often inconvenient for professionals. How easy it would be for the tailor if every man was built the same and how easy for the doctor if everyone responded to bacteria in exactly the same way. Little can be done about the fact that people differ, but it does lead us to the first 'law'[1] of treatment: *Treatment programmes should be tailored to suit each client's individual need.*

In other words one should consider the differences between people and allow one's approach to be flexible enough so that modification of a programme can be made in order to meet individual needs. Very often a treatment programme will involve more than one person. Consequently one has to think of tailoring a programme that will suit four or five different people of either sex. In this respect Ostler's words should be considered: 'It is more important to know what kind of man has a disease than what kind of disease a man has.' The philosophy behind these words will become clearer if one considers the phobic state: one client may respond to the behavioural method known as 'implosion' whereas another client with a similar phobia may become worse via such a method. The first 'law', then, suggests that the individuality of the client should always be a prime consideration. It is not sufficient simply to try to place yourself in his position, a philosophy often put forward today, since you have different standards, different norms and different stress levels. Ridiculous as it may sound, you need to put more than yourself in the client's position. Consider your own circle of friends; how different are their lifestyles from your own? Attitudes tend to be different, as do humour and artistic taste. Programmes of events with which people break up their days so that normality and predictability enter their lives, or their 'timetables', will be different.

As a practical exercise it may be worthwhile to note down the obvious differences between yourself and a friend, then consider that such differences occur within all relationships. This is the sort of attitude one should bring to the client encounter.

Our second 'law of treatment' concerns responsibility. Learning to be helpless tends to be an occupational hazard within a patient-career. One can only guard against this process by encouraging a client to take responsibility for his own treatment. Nothing appeals to many human beings more than taking a back seat and letting someone else suffer all the stress. We can be lead far better than pushed. Imagine that someone, an eccentric millionaire, entered your life and took responsibility for all your finances, expecting nothing in return. To begin with it would probably be great fun, but what would happen once you became dependent upon his financial resources? A similar situation emerges during illness: a person arrives with the skill and expertise and takes over the management of a client's life. Very often the client passively allows this situation. The trouble begins when problems arise in the absence of the professional. The client has not learned to cope, or rather has become accustomed to not getting involved and allowing others to solve the problems and make the decisions. The second 'law', then, suggests that *the majority of responsibility for treatment should be handed over to the client*. In this respect the notion that 'a client should want to get well' takes on a different meaning: a client should be actively encouraged to get well by participating in the management of his own treatment. Various strategies exist that can help to bring about this situation, some of which will be discussed later.

The third 'law' concerns the *honesty principle*. Therapeutic relationships tend to thrive and mature on honesty. It appears to be a perfect culture medium for such relationships. They can, however, be totally destroyed by one broken promise. To a certain extent, psychiatry has been guilty of making promises that it cannot keep (Skidmore and Stoker, 1974). This can produce a negative attitude in the exposed client, e.g. the client who has had a lot of experience of the psychiatric service. The results of such negative attitudes may cause a sort of 'bandwagon' or 'carousel' effect where clients drift from one type of therapy to the next without having commitment to any. The giving of truthful information, however, can influence a person's behaviour (Peterson and London, 1965). What we now find, then, is that laws two and three are interrelated since the process of giving truthful information can also illustrate that the responsibility for overcoming a problem is largely the client's (Peterson and London, 1965).

Let us recap on the three laws prior to examining each in further detail:

(1) First Law: make the treatment fit the individual.
(2) Second Law: do not take on all the responsibility yourself.
(3) Third Law: make no promises.

If we consider the first law, that treatment should be tailored to meet the individual's needs, we need to consider many things. Most texts concerning treatment appear to imply that problems conform to some kind of norm and that a package can be utilised when treating all those diagnosed as 'A' and that a different package is available for those diagnosed 'B'. One could argue that this is not even true of medical care; it is certainly less true in psychiatry. The genesis of this misconception appears to lie in the professionals' attempts to pigeon-hole symptoms into some kind of recognisable order. Marks (1970) suggests that agoraphobia is the most common presenting problem of neurosis in the UK. However, one finds that wide discrepancies exist between the professionals' interpretation of the term. Indeed, one may report that one is afraid of wide open spaces, but for what reason? Much of the evidence collected for such surveys is based on pencil-and-paper tests, tests that demand an 'all-or-nothing' response. One should remember that human emotions rarely function like the simple neurone. Consider the question: 'Are you afraid of going outside your home?' Now consider two clients answering this question. Client 'A' is afraid of leaving the home because he is terrified of open spaces. Client 'B' is afraid because he is convinced that something will happen within his home while he is out. Both may respond 'always' but for different reasons. Both may subsequently be labelled 'agoraphobics'.

Such scales also use a very suspect measure of emotion. How can one measure a feeling? One man's terror may be another man's tension. Evaluative scales offer no indication of how severe the anxiety response is, or how intense the level is compared with the response that could be considered normal. There appear to be fears common to the general population (Skidmore, 1976) which are rarely used as an intensity indicator. When an individual responds with a high level of fear towards a statement one has no measure of how abnormal that response is. However, if we know that the average response towards a statement is 'x' it can be compared to our client's response and offer information regarding the abnormality of that response. Most instruments of measurement fail to illustrate such points. Consequently one should be concerned, prior to determining treatment, not what a person is afraid of, but why and to what degree. Treatment packages designed to deal with 'what a person is afraid of' may not be compatible with why he is afraid. Let us refer back to our two 'mythical' clients and introduce the conventional approach of 'gradual exposure' to wide open spaces. For Client A this approach may be effective. For Client B it might only be effective on a journey away from the home, since the anxiety is likely to reduce during homeward journeys; indeed, no discomfort is likely to be stimulated whilst the home is still in sight.

Obviously, one is using a very overt and simple difference here; in practice the differences tend to be far more subtle. However, the cases are used to illustrate the problems associated with professionally-defined problems. One should remember the passive response of clients, who tend to agree with professional statements. When the professional suggests that Client B is afraid of wide open spaces the client is not actively being dishonest when agreeing. However, this flaw in the client-professional relationship may cause faulty foundations for treatment. For this reason this text has sought to attack the notion of 'labelling' and professional-centred therapy. Hopefully, tailoring therapeutic programmes would negate the basic flaw in the relationship and encourage both parties to get behind the statement of the problem.

It follows, then, that to tailor therapy effectively one needs to have an accurate picture of the presenting problem from the initial assessment. Furthermore, one should not accept the assessment as an absolute and should constantly question the findings. A fumbled assessment leads to fumbling treatment. Therapy can be likened to a ready-made suit: the jacket fits fine, but look at the trousers! Even a tailored suit may require some alterations.

To summarise: clients can often be lead into giving a false picture of the problem and the professional needs to know exactly what the problem is; approximations just are not good enough. A weed should be attacked at its roots; pulling off the shoots may look tidy but it is rarely effective.

It has already been suggested that laws two and three are inter-related and consequently we can consider them together. Gellerman (1974) argues that a person is more committed to a decision if he has some responsibility for that decision. Added to this is the fact that one cannot make effective decisions without the necessary information. The notion of commitment will be discussed later in its own right but it is important to mention at this stage that it is a crucial component of therapy.

Let us revert back to our imaginary clients for the purpose of examining responsibility and honesty. Responsibility is, again, a nebulous concept and is easier to assume, for some people, than evade. On the part of the professional it will, at first, take an active effort not to take all the responsibility. On the other hand, it is not something that can be handed over in package form. Clients have to be gradually eased into the role since they usually expect the professional to take a leading role in therapy. Initial steps in responsibility-sharing can be made during the information-giving process. For example, let us examine Client A. The professional has already gathered some idea of the presenting problem from the assessment and now has to proceed with treatment plans. The client's responsibility can be implied at this stage by recapping or redefining the problem: 'Can you tell me what you think is wrong with you?'

The reply may, of course, be 'nothing', in which case it may be of help to discover what the client thinks other people think is wrong with him. This type of discussion is often very valuable when the whole family is involved in the programme. We ourselves have had several experiences of such a response. In one particular case a middle-aged man refused to accept that he was even involved with the problem, his view being that every member of his family had 'changed' and hence it was their problem and for them to sort it out. He was eventually drawn into the programme because he wanted to save his marriage. However, his idea of the problem was expressed in response to the question: 'What would you say is mainly interfering with your life?'

If we consider our imaginary Client A, he might respond: 'Going outside.' This would give the professional opportunity to examine the problem further:

'What is it about going outside that disturbs you?'
'The actual space . . . it makes me feel sick and dizzy.'

It is important not to suggest symptoms to clients. If it appears that they should suffer certain symptoms from the professional's point of view, they may well adopt them. The questions should seek to draw out information and not give it. For example, the client may simply state: 'The open air bothers me.' If the professional then asks 'Does it make you feel sick and dizzy?', the client may well give an affirmative response thinking that perhaps he ought to feel sick and dizzy. Professionals can easily fall into the trap of telling a client what he or she suffers and often the client is so overawed by the occasion that he fails to challenge the assertions (Skidmore, 1980). By using non-directive questions an accurate statement of the problem is more likely to occur, that is, the client's and the family's view of the problem rather than that shaped by the professional.

Once the problem has been defined to the satisfaction of all parties the professional should lay his cards on the table. With regard to Client A something along these lines could be useful:

> You may have developed a condition which has been called agoraphobia, a morbid fear of wide open spaces. Often this fear is so intense that people suffering from it would do anything rather than go out. Would you say that that is basically true of yourself? It is important that you add to or correct anything I say during our conversations . . . you know better than me what bothers you; I can only guess what you are going through. So, unless you explain exactly how you feel about something we could all misunderstand its importance. This fear is a psychological problem, that doesn't mean that you are going mad and it is by no means unusual. (Many clients feel that they have something unique and extremely silly (Skidmore and Stoker, 1974).) Do you think you are physically ill?

This last question is important if a client has revealed the physical symptoms associated with phobic states. If the client is convinced that he is physically ill he is unlikely to develop commitment towards psychological intervention. Whether the client states that he believes he is physically ill or not, he should be given the option of confirming the notion: 'We could organise an examination by a medical doctor just to make sure.' This statement would reinforce the client's status in the relationship, in that the professional is going to act on one of his suggestions and not subtly ridicule his contributions by brushing them off with explanations. Following a medical examination the client would then want to know why he gets sick if there is nothing physically wrong with him. One should not evade explanations because they are complex; clients can be very intelligent and you will illustrate your willingness to give information by clarifying such points. Such an explanation could be:

> Well, many people with phobias get sick. You know how some people say they suffer from their nerves? Well, they're not all wrong. In our bodies we have a nerve system called the Sympathetic Nervous System, it sort of overrides the normal nerve impulses during emergencies. You know the feeling you get when you're

frightened, beating heart, quickened breathing? Well, that's the body's way of preparing you for action, more oxygen in the blood and the blood moving faster in case you need to run. Normally it is a short-lived feeling, but during prolonged stress other organs are influenced such as the stomach, in fact the whole of the digestive system. Did you ever have that pre-exam urgency of the bladder? That's a similar thing on a lesser scale to what you get now. Very often it becomes an habitual response; by that I mean you can convince yourself that you'll feel ill in a certain situation so the body obliges. Like being air-sick, if you approach the plane saying 'I bet I'll be sick, I bet I'll be sick', the chances are you will be. In that situation you convince your body that it is ill, and after a few repeat performances you start believing you are ill. In a way it's easier to accept this than a fear of open spaces; the body gives you an acceptable excuse for not confronting fearful situations. What we have to do is convince your body that it won't come to harm in these situations. Now, there are various strategies we can use; I can't promise that they will work for you, although they have worked for other people with similar conditions. Would you like to meet one of them? (This would reinforce the information that the therapy can help and that he (the client) is not unusual.) If the description of your problem is accurate, I feel very confident that something can be done about it.

Before going on to discuss the various strategies available it should be stated that the professional is only there to offer advice and that all the real work must be carried out by the client and his family. The various techniques available could then be briefly described and following this the client asked what he thinks should be done about the problem. This would effectively throw the ball back into the client's court, implying, to some extent, that he is expected to take part in the future management.

Again, it is stressed that the above is a suggested approach, not a rule of thumb. Approaches, like therapy, require modification from client to client. Language and style cannot be delivered in the same manner to every client. Honesty, however, should remain constant. When describing therapies the advantages should be mentioned along with the disadvantages. Honesty is its own reinforcer and crucial as a foundation for commitment.

Commitment

This is a reciprocal attitude in that it can only exist in a relationship if both, or all, parties are committed to the same process. It can, perhaps, be compared with enthusiasm. Remember your schooldays; the subjects you excelled at were no doubt the ones you enjoyed, or were enthusiastic about. In other words you developed commitment to those subjects. The reason this happened, apart from your own enjoyment, may have been because the teacher was also committed to that subject. He was enthusiastic about it and this reflected in his teaching method; the method communicated that enthusiasm to you. In the psychiatric arena your approach is your teaching method, the way you communicate your enthusiasm to the client. If you enter the encounter convinced that you are backing a loser the chances are that this attitude will reflect in your style and be picked up by the client. In a way it is the old 'Would you buy a second-hand car from this man?' situation. Your commitment will be reflected not only in your verbal style, but also by your non-verbal displays. If you betray that deep down you think you are banging your head on a brick wall, what chance has the client got of developing enthusiasm towards your methods? Without commitment, particularly on the client's part, therapy will be a struggle, if it ever gets off the ground. People tend to put a lot more effort into getting their own ideas, or ones they have been party to, in motion than ideas that have been handed down from another party (Gellerman, 1974); it could be argued that they automatically have a greater commitment to these ideas. The professional should, then, try to nurture commitment from the onset of the encounter and constantly strive to reinforce it. The free flow of information and honesty, feedback and shared responsibility can all aid the commitment process.

Approach

Having touched on approaches earlier we can now suggest a few 'laws' of approach to the professional-client encounter, bearing in mind the notions of honesty and commitment. The first 'law' is crucial for the philosophy of the approach and that is that one is entering an encounter with an *equal*. Obviously this can be a difficult attitude to develop when one party possesses knowledge that the other does not. Such a situation can be rectified by the free flow of information. By providing the client with as much information about his condition as is possible the ground can be set to discuss the problem on equal footing. Unless this is achieved the relationship cannot progress to one of shared responsibility.

The second approach law would be that the encounter should be conducted on a very *informal* level. This would reinforce the first law, since formality suggests leaders and followers. Introducing formal leaders into such encounters can destroy the free flow and generation of ideas crucial to 'client-centred therapy'. If formality is introduced into the client-professional relationship the client will find it quite easy to adopt a passive role. In a process where everyone's opinions are of value, any situation that stifles spontaneous contribution will be counter-productive. The introduction of informality does not necessarily require the liberal use of first names, since some clients may feel uncomfortable in such a situation. The professional must still be aware of, and respect, 'old fashioned' principles such as respect for age. Again, the application of the second law requires tailoring to meet the needs of individual clients. It should, however, respect the ideals and attitudes of everyone involved in the problem, as, indeed, most friendships do.

The third law is, perhaps, the most unpalatable. It demands *accessibility* of the professional. The professional, from the initial encounter, has to prove and maintain accessibility throughout the duration of the programme. This may even require divulging private telephone numbers. However, the whole philosophy of the approach, equal status and informality, cannot be instituted on a part-time basis. It would be very difficult even to initiate a relationship when making it known that your friendship is only available between the hours of eight and five. This can be implied by limiting accessibility.

To summarise: the laws of approach suggest that the professional should take an *equal status, informality* and *accessibility* to every client encounter.

Having introduced the concepts of approach and treatment laws it may now be pertinent to discuss the reasons why clients seek outside help for their problems. Such reasons have been mentioned in earlier chapters. It is suggested that crisis is the genesis of the majority of treatment seeking (Caplan, 1964; Davis, 1963; Marris, 1974). These authors examine crisis theory very effectively and readers are directed to their works for further information. Davis (1963) is perhaps the most useful since it studies the effect of crisis on the whole family. However, it may be useful to the flow of this text to examine briefly this issue.

It can be argued that a psychological disturbance within a family presents a crisis to that family. It has already been suggested that most relationships, including those within a family, are conservative in nature and resistive to change. A crisis, by definition, causes change. Consequently, a crisis within a relationship presents a second crisis because of the natural impulse to resist change. It is estimated that 90 per cent of psychiatric admissions are due to crisis (Caplan, 1964). But what causes the crisis? Is one man's crisis another man's irritation? Certainly people are not uniform in their reactions to adverse situations. For example, death affects everyone at some time or another; some people go completely to pieces during this type of crisis, while others maintain their stability. One could argue, then, that a crisis is not merely an adverse event; it appears to be a process that is dependent upon events, people and, perhaps, history. First of all, let us consider crises as developing on three levels:

(1) Accidental: loss or threat of loss, e.g. a death in the family.
(2) Developmental: cognitive disturbance, e.g. that which can be called 'identity-crisis' which occurs upon the almost sudden realisation that one has no direction or goal in life. This is an insidious development rather than a sudden event.
(3) Restriction: loss of liberty or incapacitated lifestyle, e.g. due to hospitalisation or paralysis.

Each one of these could cause psychological disturbance since they necessitate change and disrupt the predictive element in life. They need not necessarily occur separately and could easily overlap, so that aspects of (1), (2) and (3) occur together. We survive life, in a psychological sense, by being able to make predictions. These predictions help us to construct the timetables we use every day: we tend to break our days into sections, so that we can confidently manage ourselves. Normally, we employ various mechanisms to cope with minor problems. Our timetables are part of these mechanisms in that they tend to allow for minor disturbances and delays, a late train for instance. However, these mechanisms sometimes break down and a crisis arises, causing a protraction between point A (problem) and point B (solution). The emotion generated between these two points is usually negative: tension, uncertainty, anxiety and even panic. The more time spent between the two points the more intense the emotion becomes, and the more anxious we become the less likely we are to see the solution. It is not easy to stay calm and roll up in a rug when you burst into flames; the natural impulse would be to run like hell! It is suggested that people are more receptive to outside influence during crisis (Caplan, 1964) and it is not too difficult to see why. If people are more receptive to outside influence then it is crucial that the influence is positive. It has been argued that crisis can be habitual, if clients are not directed through it, but led through it, it may be easier for them to see less severe problems as crises.

One would further argue that a crisis is not an event peculiar to an individual. Like a vortex, it has the capacity to draw in others, particularly other family members. Let us examine a simulated case, that of a developmental crisis. The subject is a young, intelligent mother who forsook her career to raise two children. Previously she had a promising career, her own circle of friends and the interest of her work. Since her voluntary sojourn as a housewife her whole interest has been her children. The time comes when the children go to school, leaving mother alone. Her status in the children's eyes may diminish and teachers take over. The mother is left with lots of empty time on her hands, she has lost contact with many of her former friends and her prime interests now occupy themselves in the schoolroom. Suddenly she realises that she has nothing in front of her. The children can only get older and more independent, and the husband has his own life and separate interests, i.e. work and friends. She has lost contact with her former career and does not have the confidence to go back to work. She feels suddenly isolated, a small part of her husband's world, a small part of her children's world, but having no world of her own. She has the time to dwell on her situation, becomes depressed and irritable which in turn causes her external display towards her family to change. She has now changed in the family's eyes and become unpredictable. Her new display can easily be open to misinterpretation and false reasons can be ascribed to it, e.g. 'she hates us', 'she has a lover'. Her family in turn reacts to her behavioural displays, perhaps causing her to feel guilty and misunderstood. Trapped in the limbo between problem and solution she quickly loses sight of a solution and even the reason for her state. She is unable to say lucidly what is wrong with her and members of her family then feel she is keeping things from them. The crisis has now trapped them all. They all become uncertain, anxious and unable to see any solution. Without guidance and objectivity they continue to translate the events as they see them and eventually the relationships could disintegrate.

Now, labelling the wife as a depressive would not solve the problem. It could reinforce her feelings of misunderstanding and even provide some short-term relief for the rest of the family by giving reasons for the change. Such a crisis requires a family solution; the crisis must be recognised by all family members and all their efforts directed towards a solution. The mother would require reassurance regarding her place in the family and absolution from her guilt. The whole family would be required to aid her in finding a 'goal' in life; without their help she could easily continue to feel misunderstood.

It is not difficult to see how housewives can become institutionalised and suffer from all the implications that the process suggests: loss of confidence, learned helplessness and even phobias. Consequently, a great deal of support would be required on the part of the family when attempting to solve the problem. After a few years bound to the home, because of children or other dependants, a person may quickly lose the skills and confidence concomitant with a career. In the above case the depression would be a reaction to the lifestyle which may be reinforced by the faulty interplay arising in the family; in this respect it is a secondary psychological problem. Antidepressants would only be palliative and may only succeed in enforcing the 'sick-role' on the client. If the client is placed in the sick-role she may lose sight of the original problem and the family may find assurance in the fact that it need do nothing other than support her illness. Seeing the depression and nothing else is tantamount to burying the professional head in the sand.

We arrive, then, at the point where the professional must consider that he or she is likely to be involved in problems other than those of a psychiatric nature, i.e. life problems which manifest psychiatric symptoms. Crises do not automatically equate with psychiatric disturbance, although the effects of a crisis can indicate such a disturbance, particularly if one is expecting to see just this. At this stage, that is the stage when the professional realises he is not dealing with pure psychiatry, he needs to ask himself: 'Can I handle it?' In view of the rise in psychiatric community caseloads it is a logical question. Why burden your caseload with a client you cannot help? Your time is valuable to your clients; if you cannot handle the case, call in someone who can. It appears that there is another law in here somewhere.

Crises appear to have definite anatomies (Davis, 1963); certain stages occur in sequence. Briefly, these could be stated:

(1) Denial or refusal to accept that something is wrong by all or any of the persons involved; a stage which equates with the normalising stage of the deviancy-model.
(2) Recognition, the point where it has to be accepted that something is wrong, although the 'victims' may have no real idea what.

(3) Impact, the period of limbo where 'victims' are forced to accept the situation, become uncertain, and try to make sense of the situation but tend to lose direction altogether. During this stage scapegoating may occur or false reasons be ascribed so that 'sense' can be made of the situation.

It may now be useful to consider a crisis as a collection of events rather than as a single, sudden change in lifestyle. A crisis could be such a collection of events, often unrelated and singularly offering no threat, but when the events are strung together they then prove extremely threatening to those involved. Consider, for example, the case of the housewife we discussed earlier. The crisis may have been a result of the children going to school, but that event did not cause it. Rather it was the glue that stuck a collection of events together, the final straw, as it were. Let us examine her life in terms of these events:

(1) She leaves her career to care for her children.
(2) The children occupy her time and she eventually adopts their timetables: meals, toiletting, bedtime, etc.
(3) Living by her children's timetables provides her with little time to maintain her previous skills.
(4) She now moves into the mothers' circle and may well lose contact with previous friends, particularly those who are childless.
(5) Gradually her total interest is child-dominated; children become a major point of conversation in most relationships.
(6) The whole process is insidious in that she is not aware that it is happening.
(7) The children go to school.
(8) The timetable of her life is suddenly removed and predictability goes out of the window.
(9) She is suddenly thrust into an isolated timetable which gives her time to dwell on what she has lost in life.
(10) Her behaviour changes as a reaction to the sudden change.

If we consider this lady's previous lifestyle (career) as line A and her motherhood as line B we can illustrate the changes in her life as shown in Figure 5.1. The loss of the earlier lifestyle did not itself cause a crisis because it dissipated gradually and was superceded by another lifestyle

Treatment Approaches

(motherhood). Her new lifestyle (motherhood), however, terminated or changed suddenly and there was nothing to supercede it. Obviously the case is oversimplified but it does illustrate that crises need not be as sudden and dramatic as they seem. It should also be possible to observe the symptoms of an emerging crisis and train the 'victims' in crisis management before it comes to a peak. This would, obviously, only be possible within at-risk populations and clients who suffer recurring crises.

Figure 5.1: Changes of Lifestyle Precipitating Crisis (see Text for Explanation)

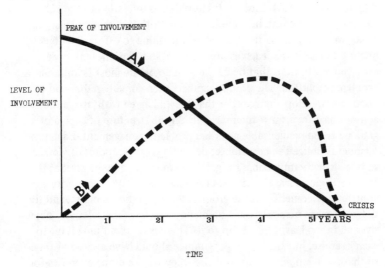

This much may be the theory, but what does one do about these problems in practical terms? First of all, remember the implications of the sick-role. Solzhenitsyn (1963) describes such effects quite succinctly: 'he'd lost the habit of planning for the next day, for a year ahead, for supporting his family. The authorities did his thinking for him about everything — it was somehow easier that way.' Bearing this sort of effect in mind let us examine various strategies that can negate the 'learned responses' associated with the clients of professionals. Primarily we should be concerned with negating avoidance behaviour and substituting the skills necessary for clients and their families to face and solve problems. Secondly we should refuse to take total responsibility and should structure therapy in such a way that total responsibility is eventually handed over to the client or family. This should be made clear to the client or family from the start: 'It's a real crisis for you, wake to it, and act. It's not so hard once you realise and begin' (Shaw, 1962).

One method that appears to have been successful in the past and that incorporates these principles is the use of consensus techniques, or decision-making games (Skidmore and Stoker, 1974). This is a structured process ideally suited for family therapy, that commences in a non-threatening way and eventually encourages groups to identify, describe and manage their own problems. A simple problem is presented on paper and is followed by a list of management options (e.g. as shown in Figure 5.2). Initially the problem is unrelated to the clients and this helps them to become familiar with the process and also discover that everyone in the group has something to offer. The object of the exercise is that each group member, in isolation, rank-orders the management options that he or she feels to be the most favourable for problem resolution. The group members then come together and by discussion develop a rank-order that they all agree with. Bargaining and compromise are against the rules. Within the structure of such a programme is the recognisable goal, i.e. problem management. Each group member is obliged to contribute, defending his own point of view, etc., so it is virtually impossible for group members to stay passive, as they are able to do in less-structured group methods. The pressure for contributing comes from the group rather than the therapist, and the therapist takes no active part; he merely describes the rules and objectives and then leaves the group to it. There is no fixed time limit to each exercise, but the whole programme should have a sense of time so that the members do not feel that they will be doing exercises for ever. The method has three clear stages:

(1) Exercises, the pencil-and-paper problems.
(2) Practice, rehearsing the skills that are taught.
(3) Action, using the skills to solve the problem.

Within the first stage there is the introductory problem, which can be professionally devised, followed by two or three problems, which may be similar to the problem shared by the group but not too similar so that issues of identification occur. These problems gradually focus more and more towards the group (see Figures 5.3 and 5.4). They can be professionally devised in the initial stages and eventually substituted for the problems devised by previous groups. The final phase of stage

Treatment Approaches

one is to encourage the group or family to place a statement of its problem on paper along with possible management options. It will have become familiar with therapeutic methods during the previous exercises when the professional explained and described the various options stated.

Figure 5.2: General Problem with Management Options

You are a member of an aircrew who has crash-landed on a tropical island. Your object is to travel 200 miles across land, due west, where you know civilisation exists. You can only travel an average 25 miles per day. The nights are intensely cold and the temperature rises to unbearable heat at midday. Out of the items listed below, rank-order them in terms of priority for survival quality. Consider first of all that you could only take one of the items with you; having eliminated that from the list select a second, and so on.

Matches, one box
Tent canvas
200 feet of tin foil
Large knife
Pistol
Magnetic compass
10kg of dehydrated milk
Life-raft
500 feet of rope
5kg of dried soup
A ball of string
10-gallon water carrier
First-aid kit
Axe

Additional information: all high ground, mountains, etc., lie to the north. The nearest ocean lies 300 miles to the south. The island measures 300 miles east-to-west and 550 miles north-to-south. You will cross reasonably level ground, but that will include jungle and desert.

Source: Rope and Skidmore (1978).

Figure 5.3: Problem with Relevance to Group Studying It

You are a member of a therapeutic team, designed to advise care on certain nervous disorders. The subject you are dealing with is a young married woman who is in danger of becoming afraid of leaving the house to the extent that she is nauseous and dizzy even when standing in the garden. Her husband is now having to take care of all external domestic chores, e.g. shopping, hanging-out washing, as well as continuing his normal employment. From the options below your task is to set, in order of preference, those most beneficial and lasting to the subject. Number the one you consider most important '1' etc.

(1) Admit her into hospital as in-patient _____

(2) Persuade her husband to divorce her _____

(3) Prescribe medication _____

(4) Treat her at home within her own environment _____

(5) Try and keep her off medication _____

(6) Get her to see a psychologist _____

(7) Bring her into hospital as out-patient or day patient _____

(8) Get her to see a psychiatrist _____

(9) Have her shopping delivered and arrange a home-help _____

(10) Encourage her to go out regularly with friends, visit relatives, etc. _____

Name _____   Group _____

Figure 5.4: Problem with Relevance to Group Studying It

This case involves a married woman in her late thirties with two teenage daughters. After the death of her father she suffers a nervous breakdown. The eldest daughter is a constant source of worry and the wife continually argues with her husband about her. The wife has tried several times to kill herself and has been in and out of hospital several times. Five weeks after the eldest daughter married she went off with her groom's eldest brother and the shock sent her mother 'into herself'. For the last six months she has been very depressed, has not been eating and speaks very little. She displays aggression by smashing things and does not appear to remember the incidents afterwards. She is very tense, withdrawn, does not go out and the marriage is gradually breaking down. The husband and remaining daughter have no idea how to cope with the situation. From the options below your task is to set, in order of preference, those most beneficial and lasting to the subject. Number the one you consider most important '1' etc.

(1) Admit her into hospital as in-patient   _____

(2) Prescribe her medication   _____

(3) Admit her to a day hospital   _____

(4) Get her to see a psychologist   _____

(5) Persuade her to go to a relaxation class   _____

(6) Send her out to work   _____

(7) Get her to see a pscyhiatrist   _____

(8) Send her out on her own   _____

(9) Try and keep her off medication   _____

(10) Treat her at home in her own environment   _____

Name _____   Group _____

The second stage would be to practise the skills needed in order to carry out the management in real life. Again, the professional would only advise and instruct rather than take an active part. In this way the clients gradually take on the responsibility. Clients involved in this type of therapy stated that they had become more honest with themselves and more self-assertive (Stoker and Skidmore, 1973). Throughout the second and third stages the group members rate themselves and each other so that feedback of progress is provided. Simple self-rating scales can be devised, based on each individual's view of his or her problem. This could be based on, for instance, inability to enter into conversation and inability to make decisions. The problems could be transcribed onto cards and be accompanied by a simple scale of success:

	Poor		Good			Very good	
Conversation	0	1	2	3	4	5	6
Decision making							

Each member of the group would keep a card for that particular client as well as the client self-rating. The cards could then be periodically compared and the client could see how his own assessment compares with that of others. The exercise would also provide the basis of useful discussion within the group. Discussion can be a useful component to all group methods, certainly when spontaneous. As a method of relaxing from the structure of the consensus method, ending each session with a period of discussion could be very productive. The discussion could initially commence with views about progress, usefulness of the method and problems encountered and gradually be directed towards less related items such as news, the price of beer, etc. The beauty of this method is that it immediately involves the group in its own treatment, and encourages decision-making and the taking of responsibility. It does not necessarily need to be confined to families, of course, since groups of individual clients or two family groups can be brought together.

Having involved the clients in their own treatment and reached a point where they admit formally that there is a problem, by putting it on paper, the time arrives when practical intervention is required. This should be a natural progression and all members should be aware of its arrival. The type of intervention would naturally depend upon the type of problem and one should not decry the use of any particular psychotherapeutic method. It can be argued that the problem with psychiatry today is that it is divided. Camps have developed within the field specialising in behaviourism, psychoanalysis, the social model and various other models. All can justifiably claim success and all can be blamed for failure. Rather than supporting any one camp it appears to be more logical to examine each model and take the good points or even apply a model direct where appropriate. These models are fully described in Siegler and Osmond (1974).

However, back to the method under discussion. The exercise might prove to be effective merely by encouraging group members to admit that they have a problem. But suppose the problem that the group defines is one of 'agoraphobia'. The professional is required to provide the necessary information regarding this 'problem' and how it can be tackled. In the behavioural context this would necessitate the group being practised in at least two methods:

(1) 'Gradual exposure', in which the client is presented with situations that become gradually more threatening, based on the client's own hierarchy. The method can be carried out in the imagination prior to *in-vivo* (real life) exposure or initiated *in vivo* at the beginning.
(2) 'Implosion', in which the client is exposed to the most threatening situation imaginable and kept there until the fear subsides.

Both methods usually incorporate the use of relaxation techniques. Consequently the group would require education about relaxation, reinforcement, constructing hierarchies and presenting fearful situations with the use of non-fearful models.

Relaxation can be a problem in itself and it can be practical to direct the whole group through a relaxation programme. Many methods of relaxation tend to rely on the client's voluntary use of a cassette tape or record that directs the relaxation technique. To be effective the technique requires daily practice, the philosophy being that once mastered it can be summoned when required, the client being able to relax at will when confronted by fearful situations. However, consider that the use of 'special' tapes and records not only lacks the human touch but also interferes with everyday life. They can draw attention to the problem in a negative manner, since the client might be required to excuse himself from the rest of the family, enter a quiet, secluded area and listen to the tape. In the real world of anxiety states this may prove to be too traumatic. Apart from drawing attention to the client's 'oddity' it also implies that special therapy is required. In our experience such taped techniques are rarely effective; when they are effective they are extremely useful but they are not everyone's choice. Many clients find it hard to participate in this kind of voluntary regime, either because they feel ridiculous or the effort of excusing themselves from the family group is too great.

Such obstacles can be overcome by tailoring the technique to the individual and making it as natural as possible. One method that appears to overcome the difficulties of relaxation therapy was by the use of music (Skidmore, 1975). Again, the client is required to participate in the planning of the method. Basically the client selects several pieces of music, in his possession, that he finds particularly relaxing. The music is then ranked in order of its relaxing quality and recorded, in sequence, on tape. The client can then be 'conditioned' to relax to the music. This would necessitate the professional 'talking' the client through the music several times. An example of this talk-through is as follows.

The client should make himself as comfortable as possible, either lying down or sitting. Once comfortable the music should be turned on, the volume being audible but low enough for the professional's voice to be heard above it. The client should then be reassured that he will not be hypnotised, nor encouraged to do anything silly and also advised not to fight against the sensations he will experience. The talk-through can then commence:

> Please concentrate on the music – let it flow over your body. Try and shut out all other noises except the music and my voice. Now, fix your gaze onto some object, a speck on the wall or anything you choose and keep staring at it, blinking as little as possible. [The professional's voice should grow progressively 'softer'.] The longer the music plays the heavier your body will feel – your eyes are feeling particularly heavy. Don't let them close yet, keep staring, hardly blinking and I'm going to count from one to five; with each number I count your whole body will get heavier still, your eyes will be so heavy that you will have to close them. When I get to five, let them close and keep them closed. One . . . concentrate on the music and my voice, all other sounds growing very distant . . . two . . . only my voice and the music clear now . . . getting heavier and heavier . . . three . . . your eyes very heavy . . . your body pressing down on the chair . . . four . . . very heavy now . . . can't keep your eyes open . . . five . . . close your eyes . . . you're feeling very heavy,

but not too uncomfortable. Now I want you to imagine something particularly pleasant, perhaps a day on the beach. It's a warm day, not too hot, just right. You've nothing at all to do today, no one to meet, just the whole day to relax. You can feel the warmth of the day spreading over your body. You are aware of nothing other than the music and my voice and the heavy warmth. In the distance you can perhaps hear the cry of a gull or the lapping of the ocean on the beach; other than that, it's very still, quiet and comfortable. So comfortable that you sink deeper and deeper into this feeling, the music washing over you . . . your body pressing into the chair . . . heavier and heavier. Now, I'm going to count from one to five again, and with each number I count all the heaviness will gradually leave your body. Think of yourself as a sand-filled rag-doll . . . there are holes in your feet and the sand is running through the holes. Starting at your head you will feel lighter and lighter as the sand leaves through your neck, chest, stomach, down through your legs and out onto the floor. As it leaves you feel lighter and lighter. It's a very pleasant feeling, all the heaviness and tension leaving you. Keep breathing steadily, nothing to worry about . . . at the count of five you'll not feel your body at all, it will be so light . . . only aware of my voice and the music, warmth . . . quiet. One . . . all the weight starting to go . . . leaving your head now. It is taking all the tension with it . . . two . . . head very light . . . all the weight, the heaviness draining into your chest . . . all the tension going . . . three . . . stomach getting very light . . . heaviness and tension entering your legs . . . four . . . very slowly, from the top of your legs the lightness is driving the heaviness away . . . past your knees . . . the sand trickling through your feet onto the floor. Very light . . . five . . . listen to the music and my voice . . . all weight gone now . . . gentle, quiet, warm, relaxed. Every time you listen to this music it will become easier and easier to get to this state . . . every time you hear the music you will feel relaxed . . . no tension . . . just this warm relaxed feeling. Still not light enought yet, there's still some heaviness there . . . concentrate on my voice and the music . . . you are going to get lighter still. Think about your breathing . . . I want you to breathe a bit deeper than normal to the rhythm I'm going to establish now . . . when I count one . . . I want you to breathe in, deeply . . . on two, hold your breath and three breathe out, all the way out. [Make sure not to interrupt the natural rhythm and count one at the point of natural inspiration.] One . . . breathe in . . . two, hold it . . . the air catching those last pieces of heaviness . . . three, breathe out, all the way out ... more weight leaving you with that air ... One .. every breath making you lighter ... two ... lighter and lighter ... three ... all the tension going. [Repeat several times.] Now breathe normally again ... you are very light now ... so light that if I were to fix a balloon to your body it would just float up after that balloon ... no weight, no tension ... very relaxed, very warm and as long as the music plays you'll feel even more relaxed. Every time you hear this music it will be easier to reach this stage ... relaxed and warm ... no worries, nothing to disturb you. Concentrate on the music and the pleasant scene you can imagine in front of you ... listen to my voice ... very relaxed ... warm ... every time you hear the music you will feel relaxed.

Now I'm going to count down from five to one ... and with each number I count you will feel more and more alert, more awake ... until you are fully alert, fully awake ... but still relaxed. Five ... starting to feel the chair again ... normal weight coming back ... four ... feeling a little alert now [louder] ... three ... feeling alert, awake, but relaxed [louder and harsher] ... two ... more and more awake ... eyes opening ... one ... fully alert, open your eyes. Stay where you are for a few moments and enjoy the relaxed feeling!

It may be useful at this stage to have a chat with the client about the exercise. Some of the stages may need to be repeated at first and the first session usually takes much longer than subsequent sessions. The technique is semi-hypnotic, which is why the client should be talked out of it. Again, remember that this talk-through is only an example and the practical technique will require modification from client to client. It may help if the client describes a pleasant scene to you prior to the exercise, just in case you accidentally hit on one of his fears — some clients may be afraid of the sea, for instance.

The advantage of the technique is that the client does not need to draw attention to himself to practise, for it is quite a normal social activity to listen to music. Indeed, the whole family could be involved, and a responsible family member could even talk another through it. The other major advantage is that the client has helped to design the exercise in that he chose the music.

Once the client has been 'conditioned' by the process, two or three sessions often being sufficient, the music can be used during the therapeutic sessions, rather than one expecting the client to relax at will. The music can be played from the onset of the session so that the client is relaxed from the very beginning. Let us now use a long suffering

Treatment Approaches 87

spider-phobic as an example. After discussion the client has produced a hierarchy of situations and opted for the gradual exposure method. The professional has obtained a collection of 'spidery' threats. The family is present and has volunteered and been briefed to act as non-fearful models. The seating has been arranged in the circular mode:

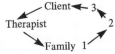

The therapist switches on the music at low volume and explains that he has a collection of objects which he is going to pass around the room anti-clockwise. He instructs the client and the family to observe exactly what he does with them and asks them to repeat his actions. The objects are all based on the client's own hierarchy:

Most fearful	Handling a large live spider	1
	As above, but in jar	2
	As above, but jar has screw top	3
Fearful	Handling large dead spider	4
	As (2) with dead spider	5
	As (3) with dead spider	6
	Handling small live spider	7
	As (7) in jar	8
	As (7) in screw-top jar	9
	Handling small dead spider	10
	As (10) in jar	11
	As (10) in screw-top jar	12
Slightly fearful	Handling plastic spider	13
	Handling spider-like objects	14
	Looking at pictures of spiders	15

The session starts with object 15, a picture of a spider. The therapist describes the object, picks it up and says: 'Look at the colours... count its legs... really look at it.' He runs the picture through his hands and touches his face with it, then passes it to the first model. It is passed around in this manner and reinforcement, i.e. approval, is offered to each person carrying out the task. The modelling is important, since it is the way that normal behaviour is learned and illustrates to the client that those carrying out the task come to no harm. The same process is carried out for each of the hierarchy items. Number 14 could be a tomato stalk; from a distance they are quite spider-like. The transition from 11 to 10 can be effectively made by passing the spider from jar to hand and back again. However, number 9 may require more detailed steps since here one is dealing with the 'real McCoy'. It is often useful to have the client touch the hands of the person who holds the jar prior to taking the object (Figure 5.5). This tends to remove the object slightly and the client can take his own time to approach it.

Figure 5.5: Touch Prior to Transfer of Object

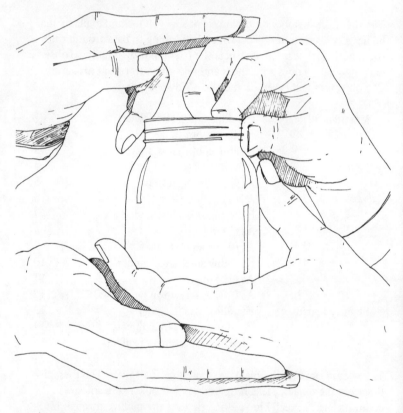

This approach would require planning with the client, but to give an example assume we have a dead spider in a screw-top jar with the top removed. The client feels a little tense with this arrangement, despite the music. The therapist models the passing-on routine by holding the jar in one hand, as above and grasping the rim between his finger and thumb. The person to receive the jar then places his hand over the therapist's and gradually moves them closer (see Figure 5.6). Gradually

the next person takes the jar and it is passed on. Next time round the
fingers are placed deeper into the jar until the spider is touched. Then
it is shaken out onto the palm. Approval should be given at every stage.
The next item on the hierarchy should not be tackled until the previous
stage is comfortably carried out by the client. Again, it is impossible to
place a time-scale on this type of therapy. Some clients may go through
the entire hierarchy in one session, others may take many sessions.
Regardless of time, the client should complete the entire hierarchy if
the phobia is to be conquered and this should be impressed on the client.

Figure 5.6: Transfer of Object

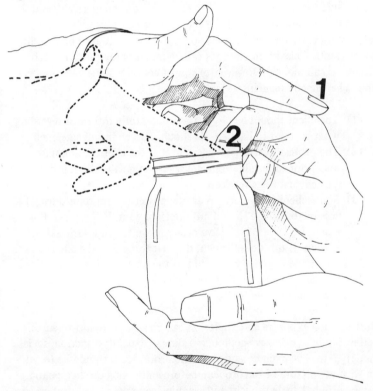

He should also be made aware that the last stage of the hierarchy
should be as ridiculous as it sounds. In other words it is important that
he handles a large spider (as long as it isn't dangerous). Although people
don't normally go around with huge spiders trotting up and down
their arms, in the case of the phobic Murphy's Law (expect the worse!)

rules. It is possible that the client completes only that part of the programme where he handles small spiders and yet feels himself to be 'cured'. But the next night, as he sits in bed, a rather large spider leaps onto his face, just to test him, and he is immediately resensitised. Consequently, in every programme of this nature the professional should be prepared for all eventualities.

The feedback process can also be incorporated into this programme by keeping the hierarchy on display and marking off each stage as it is effectively carried out. The client can then see at a glance just how he is getting along.

Having discussed gradual exposure, let us briefly consider implosion. This would involve going straight to number 1 on the hierarchy and probably use more than one large spider. This process can be very successful providing the client is kept in the situation until he is feeling comfortable. Relaxation methods can be incorporated into the techniques, as can models. However, one must consider some very important points before commencing:

(1) The client should be physically fit and fully informed regarding what is about to happen. He should also be in full agreement.
(2) The professional must be certain that the client feels comfortable prior to termination, and assured that the client is not 'acting' just to gain release.
(3) Some clients may develop drastic physical symptoms during the session, but these should not interfere with the progress. For example, some clients have been known to faint during the session. If this does happen, the first thing that the client sees when opening his eyes should be the object of his fear. If this is not carried out, fainting could be adopted as an effective avoidance technique.

Both gradual exposure and implosion can be applied to most neurotic states: phobias, obsessive-compulsive states, sexual dysfunction, social anxiety, etc. The main objective for the professional should be to get an accurate picture of the problem before embarking on therapeutic intervention. A little thought and planning can save a great deal of effort. Free discussion is seen as a valuable part of any therapy, and for this reason this text does not condemn any particular psychotherapeutic method. The relationships that can be developed under a psychoanalytical regime can be of great help. People benefit from talking about their problems.

Treatment Approaches

The techniques discussed so far are not limited for use on the neuroses. Rope (1978) successfully applied a mixture of techniques to a client diagnosed as a chronic psychotic. Again the principle of family involvement was adhered to, an accurate picture of the problem obtained and a lot of discussion used. The client in question continually disrupted her family's lives by entering into frequent conversations with God. The family eventually started to 'shun' her and refused to take her outside the home. The client retaliated by abusive and sometimes destructive behaviour inside the home. Eventually, the family considered institutionalisation as their only recourse. The client was finally admitted to an institution, which resulted in further bad behaviour. The client became abusive to staff, frequently left the hospital and would turn up at home in a hostile state. After lengthy discussions with the client Rope found that she was willing to co-operate in a programme that may lead to her discharge. She was resentful of the fact that she had been 'forced' into hospital and did not like taking medication. She did, however, accept that her family did have justification for its action. By discussing the problem with the family and client, it was discovered that the major problem stemmed from the 'holy conversations'. A contract was devised whereby the client agreed to co-operate in a programme for certain rewards. A baseline of holy conversations was taken. As the number of conversations reduced certain privileges were awarded to the client: spending a day with the family, spending a weekend at home, going out with the family and eventually day care and discharge. Everyone involved in the case was briefed regarding the programme. The ward staff would initiate conversation with the client; whenever she mentioned her 'holy conversations' they would look away, count to ten and then resume the conversation as though nothing had happened. If the client resorted to holding a conversation with God in full view of the ward, she was deliberately ignored. The programme sounds very simple, but it seemed to work. The undesired behaviour disappeared quite rapidly and the patient was discharged. Rope makes no claims of having eradicated the hallucination-delusion process and indeed it may only have been suppressed by the conscious effort of the client. However, whatever the cause the client was able to return to her family again. Perhaps Tuke displayed incredible insight back in the nineteenth century when he suggested appealing to the rational side of asylum inmates. Indeed, Rope (1978) suggests that many expressions of delusional thought are more attempts at attention-seeking than betrayals of symptoms.

It could be argued that by giving a client responsibility for his treatment one is appealing to his rational side. The treatment technique we have discussed so far places the professional in more of an advisory capacity than that of an active intervenor. He, the professional, has taken the role of guide, directing a client through his problem. Other methods of treatment can be delivered in the same or similar fashion, giving the client responsibility. Hopefully it will provide the client with that necessary 'gestalt' that will help him to manage future problems in his own right. Surely this should be the ultimate aim of intervention psychiatry? One of the more obvious methods that can be incorporated in treatment that embraces these principles is that of biofeedback. There are several devices available today that can prove very useful in therapy. Consider the myograph, the device that measures muscle tension. Clients can be taught to relax successfully with this device, but more relevant, they can be shown that many of their symptoms are the result of tension. That insight in itself may go a long way towards developing commitment towards therapy.

Let us now consider some of the other 'problems' that the professional is likely to encounter in the community. Many problems are likely to call on his or her skills as a counsellor and 'educator' rather than skills as a therapist, if indeed such skills can be segregated. Bringing objectivity to an encounter can be therapeutic in its own right, as can increasing the client's knowledge. For example, even in today's 'presumed' sexually enlightened society many cases of sexual dysfunction arise. Beware of the label! Like agoraphobia it is in danger of becoming an in-vogue diagnosis. Experience in this area may illustrate that many 'so called' dysfunctions are the result of ignorance rather than inability. Consider the following case, which is based on fact.

A couple in their early thirties were referred, initially because of the wife's agoraphobia. (Many clients with this type of personal problem will 'feign' a more common complaint and mention the real problem as though it is incidental.) The psychiatrist discovered the true nature of the problem after several sessions and referred the couple to the sexual counselling clinic. There, the couple's definition of the problem was that suddenly, after seven years of marriage, Mrs Client had developed frigidity. They had three children, were both fairly intelligent, had had normal childhoods and cared for their children. The relationship was deteriorating because of the problem; Mrs Client felt her husband's sexual demands were unreasonable and Mr Client felt that his wife did not care for him anymore. After discussion it soon became apparent that both were quite ignorant about sex. Mrs Client had been brought up to think that anything to do with genitals was filthy, except for childbirth. She washed her whole body both before and after sex. Mr Client was equally ignorant and had developed the belief that sex was a man's game. Only men got enjoyment out of it, women were always 'turned on' but never enjoyed it. In all other respects the marriage was sound and both parties were committed to its survival.

What the therapist in this case was confronted with was a two-fold problem — first of all the couple's ignorance and attitudes regarding sex and secondly the wife's, now almost hysterical, reactions towards her husband's approaches. She became very tense, even if he held her hand. A programme of education was commenced immediately; this involved attending talks about sex and discussion groups with other couples. This proved to be the hardest part, for Mrs Client refused to believe that anyone indulged in sex other than via the missionary position. Mr Client became quite abusive and almost physical when asked whether he ever 'stimulated' his wife. He felt the whole idea to be perverse. However, after several informative talks, which were reinforced in the group session, they became quite receptive to the idea. Once their attitudes had been modified a programme was instituted to counteract Mrs Client's now habitual tense reaction to her husband's approaches. The programme was based on a gradual exposure (no pun intended) regime. Mr Client agreed to sit with his wife and restrict his contact to placing his arm about her shoulders. After three days, Mrs Client agreed to return her husband's approach with a cuddle, but he would not take this any further. From there contact was built up to kissing, naked contact and finally nature took its course.

The actual method of therapeutic intervention was one of response-reward, but the main point about this case was that ignorance was the dominant factor. This was another case of a secondary problem being elevated to primary importance. If the clients' knowledge had not been improved about sex it is highly unlikely that the intervention techniques would have been successful.

There are cases of a similar nature when the problem is merely the reflection of a tired relationship. In such cases intervention is inappropriate. There are also cases where intervention may seem inappropriate but where some progress can be made. Cases of child abuse and wife abuse are such cases. Child abuse is particularly worrying since one is concerned for the child's safety. One can offer no absolute guidelines in this area; it can be argued that not to intervene is unethical and yet to intervene with no hope of success is a threat to other clients. But intervention can be successful — let us consider the following, again a case based on fact.

Jenny is a married lady in her late twenties. She has three children. The first and last child are very well-treated, but the middle child, a girl (the others are boys) is abused. She referred herself for advice because she feared injuring the child. On interview she stated that she had herself been abused as a child and that she was the only child of professional parents. She was separated from her middle child at birth on and off for the first year. The child was premature and kept in isolation for three months, and the mother was then ill for several months. The child now seemed to do all the things that irritated her mother, but the client confessed that she gave the child little attention at other times. She said that she wished it had been another boy, since she knew how to deal with boys. The therapist in charge of this case decided that one of the problems was that the mother did not have an effective model for mothering this child. Her parents had been her only model for raising girls and they beat her. Again, the child was only being given attention when abused and now demanded that attention. These points were discussed with the client who felt that they were fair comment. She felt that it might help if she saw other mothers coping with their daughters, and this was arranged. She also agreed to ignore the child during her 'demanding' phases and offer attention, in the form of affection, during quieter moments. The child was also put into play-school for three half-days a week to lessen the pressure on her mother. The programme proved effective after ten weeks and the incidence of abuse terminated.

This, simplified, case was only one success. There were failures, as there are in many instances of intervention. However, it does appear that a large amount of education was again involved in the therapeutic regime. One could argue that this is the direction that psychiatry should take. Most branches of the health caring services, certainly in the West, are too motivated by illness rather than health. It seems absurd that the public should be prompted by problems to seek guidance when these could be avoided by early education. Unfortunately, should we adopt such a programme it would start too late for many people, those who have already learned 'bad behaviour'. The other major difficulty appears to lie in the 'caring' professions' organisation: we appear to be too concerned with short-term planning. If we adopted an educational approach to psychiatry, which could prevent many problems occurring in the future, we would not see immediate results and would still be required to carry on the present system until our educated population 'came of age'. For many professionals, this makes the concept of 'prevention' unviable. Nevertheless, as professionals it seems that we have to develop a philosophy which allows the client to take the responsibility for solving problems and gives the client access to the necessary information to make this possible. In this respect the professional must change direction and move away from the giving of treatment towards the educational model. This philosophy appears to work quite well in the East, where doctors spend most of their time educating the public and only get payment providing a client remains healthy.

The present models of psychiatry appear to be symptom-orientated. Indeed, some behaviourists would argue that the cause is not important providing the symptoms can be dealt with. One could counter-argue that dealing with symptoms is purely palliative as long as the cause remains. Consider addiction; many addicts certainly respond to various types of intervention that attempt to 'get them off their stuff'. Many of those that respond subsequently resort to new stuff. This situation is revealed in the following case of an alcoholic.

A 42-year-old housewife with two children, both in their teens, self-referred following a long history of whisky-abuse. Her drinking was confined to the home and commenced some six years previously because she became lonely and depressed. She had no hobbies, few friends and her husband was away from the home a great deal for business reasons. Her drinking did not present any financial difficulties but she became worried about her health when her consumption had risen to three full bottles a day. She commenced her drinking about 9.00 a.m., as soon as she was left alone in the home, and drank steadily through the day. She had tried to resolve the problem herself, but became irritable and felt ill the longer she went without her drink.

Following medical investigation it was discovered that her physical health was, indeed, starting to suffer and she was referred to the psychology department of the hospital. After discussion she agreed to be admitted for three days to undergo intensive aversion therapy. The programme devised was quite horrific but even after a full explanation she consented to co-operate. For the three days of the programme she was isolated in a single room. The room was lavishly decorated with whisky posters, bottles and, after much effort, a permanent aroma of whisky. She was flung straight into the programme at 9.00 a.m. on the first day with an injection of apomorphine (a strong emetic) and allowed to drink whisky as she wished. The resulting vomit was not removed, so that after a time it overflowed onto the floor. The 'degradation' was reinforced by non-verbal cues from the staff in attendance, who were briefed to act disgusted when entering the room, but to say nothing. The 'punishment' was reinforced by periodic electric-shock aversion. This was carried out by a regular therapist, who wired the client by her ankles, and had her sit in a chair where she attempted to consume a large tot of whisky. The therapist observed via a 'peep-hole' arrangement and delivered a shock every time the client actually tried to swallow the whisky. Consequently, more whisky ended its days on the wall, floor and client's clothing than actually found its way into the client's stomach. By the end of the second day the client was physically exhausted, retched at the sight and smell of whisky and swore never to touch another drop. The room was subsequently cleared and liberally douched with fresh-air sprays so that the client could spend the night and following day 'resting'.

During the first follow-up appointment the client was 'whisky-free' but complained of depression. She was reassured that this was a normal symptom of withdrawal. During the second follow-up, three weeks after the treatment, she was visibly depressed and again reassured. She still maintained that she could not face whisky and this was proved when she actually vomited after being offered a 'tot'. Five weeks after treatment she was far more cheerful and said she felt more like her old self. In fact she was indeed her old self, having discovered that vodka did not respond to her habitual aversion. After eight weeks, she was consuming three bottles of vodka a day and had been referred to another therapist.

The above case was written off as a failure by the therapist and the other professionals involved. However, the therapy was not a failure, for it succeeded in its objective by averting her from whisky. The failure resulted from the symptom-orientation of the regime. It ignored the fact that the client drank for a reason and consequently terminated too soon. If the therapist had gone further following his primary intervention and attacked the root of the problem, it may have been a different story. One could argue that alcohol is yet another avoidance technique. Whilst under its influence the problems appear to be insignificant. It is illogical to snatch away an individual's crutch and put nothing in its place. People avoid problems because they cannot cope with them, and removing the tactic of avoidance, the skill they have developed to 'cope', does not remove the problem. When discussing phobia-programmes we suggested going to ridiculous levels with the giant spiders, because merely removing the symptom was not enough. Professionals need to go beyond symptoms, beyond problems and provide the client with the necessary motivation and skills to solve that problem. The alcoholic described above may have been in a similar position to the housebound housewife described earlier. The former resorted to alcohol, while the housewife with the crisis only got as far as changing her behavioural display.

Hopefully, this text has been leading you to the conclusion that a client is more than the sum total of his symptoms. Treatment should accordingly be geared to consider more than symptoms. Furthermore, his problem is unlikely to affect only him and when others are affected further problems can develop. For these reasons it is suggested that treatment techniques adopt a new philosophy and encompass the principles of education and responsibility-sharing if they are to be successful. There are many texts that describe intervention techniques in detail and on the whole these are very valuable to the professional. However, one would stress that a client's outcome can only be as good as his professional's input. It is immaterial how sound a therapeutic programme is if the approach that brings it to an encounter is unsound. Only the professional can control and manage the approach and an effective approach can only come from recognising the individuality of his clients.

Note

1. The term 'law' is intended merely to provide a focus for ideas. Often, a single phrase can imply paragraphs of philosophy and consequently help to develop ideas and provide insight. The term is not intended to mean 'this is the truth, the only way to approach this subject'.

References

Caplan, G. (1964) *Principles of Preventive Psychiatry* (Tavistock, London)
Davis, F. (1963) *Passage Through Crisis* (Bobbs-Merrill, Indianapolis)
Gellerman, S. (1974) *Behavioural Science in Management* (Pelican, Harmondsworth, Middlesex)
Marks, I. (1970) *Fears and Phobias* (Heinemann, London)
Marris, B. (1974) *Loss and Change* (Routledge and Kegan Paul, London)
Peterson, D.R. and London, P. (1965) 'A Role for Cognition in the Behavioural Treatment of a Child's Eliminative Disturbance' in Ullman, L.P. and Krasner, L. (eds.) *Case Studies in Behavioural Modification* (Holt, Rinehart and Winston, New York)
Rope, J. (1978) 'The Use of Behavioural Psychotherapy with Psychotic Patients' (Unpublished research report)
Shaw, R. (1962) *The Hiding Place* (Penguin, Harmondsworth, Middlesex)
Siegler, M. and Osmond, H. (1974) *Models of Madness, Models of Medicine* (Macmillan, New York)
Skidmore, D. (1975) 'Mood Music', *New Psychiatry, 2, 19*, 17-18
—— (1976) 'Measuring Fear', *Nursing Mirror, 143, 12*, 68-9
—— (1980) 'The Hidden Machine', Microfiche *Verus* (Bournemouth, England)

Skidmore, D. and Stoker, M.J. (1974) 'Space Age Therapy', *New Psychiatry*, 1, 4, 15-16

Solzhenitsyn, A. (1963) *One Day in the Life of Ivan Denisovich* (Gollancz, London)

Stoker, M.J. and Skidmore, D. (1973) 'Report on Consensus Group Methods' (Unpublished report)

6 PROGRAMME PLANNING AND EVALUATION

Programmed Planning

One of the most confusing aspects of care is that there is often no way of identifying who is responsible for what in any given case. There may well be up to six care agents involved in some cases with no clear idea of who is trying to help with what, where one person's role ends and that of another begins. It is as well to appreciate that role-blur is vital to all care-giving and that where tasks are clearly delineated with a 'no trespassing' policy in operation, patients may fall down the middle into problem areas which are considered to be always another person's province and are therefore unaccounted for in the master plan.

As a disorder progresses and its treatment develops, there is a change in the levels of involvement of those concerned with the patient. Using an approach developed by Henderson (1966), an example is shown in Figure 6.1 of a man suffering from depression, being admitted to hospital and then discharged to the care of relatives and care-givers in the community.

Figure 6.1: Levels of Involvement with the Patient

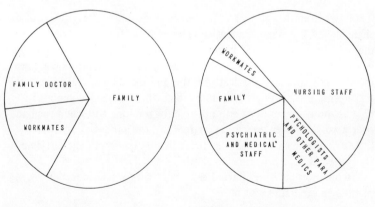

(a) Prior to Admission   (b) During Admission

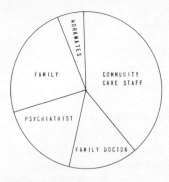

(c) Upon Discharge

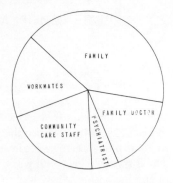

(d) Four Weeks From Discharge

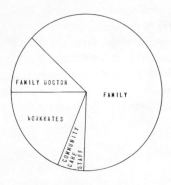

(e) Three Months Following Discharge

It follows from this that a planned programme must take account of the changing levels of involvement, and a conscious effort be made to shift the onus for care from the helping agents on to those best placed to give it, namely back to the patient and his family. Not all families will have the strengths and skills to deal with this and the time of intervention of care-agents will be longer with them than with others. The tendency may be, however, to hang on to people for too long and when the handover occurs between the caring services and the patient and his family, little or no preparation has been made in anticipation of the self-help skills needed.

Two important issues have thus been raised for consideration when planning a programme of care:

(1) The changing levels of involvement that people have with a patient and his family.
(2) The need for early involvement of the patient and his family in

anticipation of the 'handover' period.

A third aspect must also be highlighted, namely that of *time-scales*.

In general medicine it is possible to forecast with some accuracy the amount of time needed to cater for a variety of physical disorder; fractured limbs, vein stripping, tonsillectomies and metacarpal decompression for example can all be treated, cared for post-operatively and rehabilitated within a set number of weeks (given the right circumstances). What of mental disorder, can it too be placed in a tidy compartment? Almost always the answer is no. Assumptions and ideas as to how long a disorder should last abound amongst care-givers. The whole area unfortunately is grossly under-researched and often only vague feelings of unease that a case is dragging on too long, give the caring-agents the impetus to reorganise their programmes. There is evidence to show that approaches to care change the longer a case goes on and there may be a temptation to label someone as a 'chronic' rather than as an 'acute' case the longer the time of involvement lasts. Not only do the labels change but the approaches to the patient and the time spent with them change also (Butterworth, 1981). This change is based on time-scales only, and does not bear any relationship to the amount of progress that has been made (or not been made) along the road to recovery.

A fourth area for consideration is that of *goal-setting*. If a programme plan is organised how should it be phrased so that it is a useful tool and not just another piece of paper to add to an already overworked care-agent? There are two items which can be considered: aims and objectives.

Aims provide a broad description of what a care programme seeks to achieve in the long run. Aims can be useful or totally meaningless. For example, which of the following two aims would you choose for organising a programme of care for an institutionalised schizophrenic man who has just been discharged to the community after 16 years in hospital?

(1) To restore to full mental and physical health as soon as possible. He is to reintegrate into the community and participate fully as one of its members.
(2) To reintegrate as far as possible into the community within the limitations of his decreased coping skills. These skills are to be expanded as far as time, resources and the client will allow.

The two aims outlined are difficult enough, but of the two the former may be setting out to accomplish the impossible; it is arguable whether 'we normal' people can even fulfil the demands as laid out in the first aim! The second aim is more down to earth. It realises the frailties of the human being and makes an allowance for less than total success. It also gives room for the nature of the individual and his response to care.

A second example, which is again drawn from an actual case, can be given. Which of the following can be considered as a programme aim suitable for an elderly confused woman of 70 years with evidence of arterio-sclerotic changes? She is repeatedly readmitted for bizarre behaviour and is about to be discharged to the community once more.

(1) To return to the community and lead as independent a life as possible with emphasis upon resocialisation and prevention of readmission to hospital.
(2) To return to the community for the moment and live with such suitable support services as are available until her behaviour warrants some kind of intervention which is to be determined at that point in time.

The first aim presupposes that the emphasis must be upon 'discharge and be damned' usually with the person reappearing as an urgent readmission. The second aim realises that readmission is not only possible but very likely and gives room for manoeuvre. It does not draw a black-and-white division between discharge and admission (sometimes seen as success and failure) and makes no prescriptive statement as to what steps should be taken when action is needed again. This flexibility allows such action as is most appropriate to be taken at the time.

An aim provides an outline for a programme and gives it form; however it does not tell you how to accomplish the end result. It is necessary to compartmentalise activities further and provide objectives for a care programme so that not only the path is outlined but also the signposts are there to show us the way and the milestones are up to tell us how far we have come.

Objectives can be used as both signposts and milestones and state in behavioural terms what is to be achieved at a given point in time. The pursuit of objectives can be a tiresome business and if not used with discretion can lead to an inflexible programme which races headlong towards goals with prescribed time limits, thus confining the patient and his family to a tight schedule. Two objectives are given below which illustrate that it is possible to allow flexibility into a defined programme.

(1) Patient to demonstrate to the care-giver in four weeks' time the development of his budgeting skills by (i) opening a bank account, (ii) apportioning funds to pay for bills or (iii) paying an agreed alimony payment.
(2) For two weeks the patient will complete a behaviour checklist chart demonstrating the time and duration of behaviour previously defined by the nurse and the patient as ritualistic.

Objectives provide a means to an end, in that they describe what should (a) be taking place over a period of time or (b) have taken place by a specified point in time. Examples of (b) are as follows.

(1) In one week's time the patient will have decreased by 50 per cent his ritualised hand-washing, using techniques in conjunction with the care-giver.
(2) In eight weeks' time the patient will be in regular receipt of prescribed medication through (i) self dosage, (ii) witnessed receipt of same by family, (iii) weekly support visits by care-giver.

Thus it becomes possible to organise a programme of care which has not only an outline (aim) but also set routes to follow (objectives) and which consequently can be evaluated over given periods of time.

To recap, four main areas have been considered which are of importance in planning a programme of care:

(1) Changing levels of involvement that care-givers, patient and family will have one with another.
(2) The need for early and continuing involvement of the patient and family in anticipation of their taking over responsibility.
(3) The danger of using time-scales only, as a means of rating success or failure.
(4) The use of aims and objectives as a means to giving a care programme form and substance.

With these contingent points in mind we can now give some thought to the formalisation of a programme of care. This may best be done through a number of case-studies, which are here shortened for the sake of brevity.

Case Study One

Presentation

Mrs Z, a 45-year-old woman, is presented to the care team with a long and involved psychiatric history punctuated with numerous visits to hospital for stays as an in-patient. Her presenting complaint is one of depression and low self-esteem. She is childless and has a close relationship with her husband, but is seldom intimate with him. There is no other family. On each previous occasion following discharge she has immediately discontinued her medication and returned home to solitude in her house. Previous attempts at day care have proved fruitless as she refuses to leave the house. She rarely demonstrates suicidal ideas but when readmitted to hospital is in a state of agitated/confused anxiety.

Current Problems

(1) The Patient. This lady is about to be discharged into the community once more and the circle is about to repeat itself yet again. She has no more coping skills now than when she was admitted for care.

(2) The Team. The care team is faced with a problem which from previous experience is likely to be reappearing upon the doorstep very soon. Either the same approach is taken or a new method is tried which may change the present circumstances, otherwise the patient's and the team's expectations become a self-fulfilling prophesy.

The Decision

A decision is made to take a problem-solving approach and to involve the patient from the start. She agrees to this idea as no one is more tired of her current lifestyle than she! After discussions and interview with the psychiatrist, social worker and community nurse separately, all four (including the patient) meet together to devise a strategy, through problem identification.

The Problems

There are essentially four problem areas:

(1) There is always a lack of continuity of care following discharge. From being the centre of attention on the ward one day, Mrs Z is alone and isolated at home the next.
(2) Mr Z has little apparent enthusiasm for assisting his wife to get

well again. Upon exploration it is found that he has not been interviewed for two years and therefore not asked about his thoughts and views.
(3) Mrs Z discontinues her medication knowingly, thereby consciously making a decision which she knows will contribute at least in part to her return to hospital.
(4) Mrs Z has never formed a truly therapeutic relationship with any of the team and has never therefore had chance to express her true feelings about the various facets involved. She indicates a willingness to foster such a relationship and chooses the community nurse as her choice of confidante.

The Plan

Again this has four aspects:

(1) Medication will be monitored by the community nurse upon Mrs Z's discharge and supplies replenished by the patient's family doctor.
(2) The community nurse will form a working relationship with Mrs Z and work with her on (i) her inability to cope with her daily routine while on her own and (ii) giving her some chance to express her hidden feelings and difficulties.
(3) The social worker will contact the elusive Mr Z and endeavour to interview him and then find out his current position in the scheme of things.
(4) The psychiatrist will see Mrs Z every two weeks for the next six weeks and liaise with her family doctor.

In six weeks' time there will be a team (and family) evaluation of the current situation.

The Proceedings

Medication was regularly maintained but the establishment of a confiding relationship between the community nurse and Mrs Z was not proceeding as well as was initially hoped. Mrs Z could not break down her strong resistance against being able to open up to anyone.

Mr Z was interviewed by the social worker who found him to be shut out of the whole system. The things which were happening to his wife were, he felt, beyond his control and therefore he had withdrawn from any active participation in her 'ill life'. He was currently impressed by the fact that Mrs Z was regularly taking medication and offered (eventually) to participate in the next team meeting.

The Six Week Evaluation

A team meeting was convened and attended by all participants including Mr and Mrs Z. After discussion both with and without Mr and Mrs Z problems were identified and decisions were reached about their proposed resolution.

Problem A. Mrs Z has been treated in isolation from her husband and he has indicated a willingness to participate. Resolution: conjoint therapy once per week will be undertaken by Mr and Mrs Z, the community nurse (M) and the social worker (F). Aims: (i) to promote Mr Z's capacity to assist his wife when she is anxious and depressed, and (ii) to move the onus for care and the confiding relationship back to the marriage setting.

Problem B. Taking of medication. Resolution: Mrs Z should be tested for her capacity to self-dose with medication and the community nurse should withdraw from this aspect when satisfied that medication is being taken. Aim: to allow Mrs Z to take responsibility for self-dosage of medication.

Problem C. The family doctor feels he is not being sufficiently informed as to the current state of Mrs Z. Resolution: the psychiatrist will write to and the community nurse will go and see the family doctor. Aim: to see if the family doctor can offer any further information or advice on the Zs.

A further evaluation will be undertaken by the team in six weeks' time.

The Twelve Week Evaluation

A team meeting was held and a number of decisions were reached.

Problem A. Weekly conjoint therapy is now well established and will continue for the next three months. There will be a phased withdrawal by the therapists after this point in time should evaluation at this time prove to be satisfactory.

Problem B. Mrs Z has demonstrated her ability to self-medicate and will take responsibility for this from now on.

Problem C. The family doctor is now happy with his knowledge of the current situation and, although not actively involved apart from prescribing medication, will continue to be informed on a monthly basis.

Further evaluation would take place in three months' time.

Comments

By systematically organising a programme of care with a problem-solving approach it has become possible to deal to good effect with a somewhat difficult case. Although a team approach was taken, one essential member had been left out — the family doctor. When this deficit was made good, the case progressed without too many difficulties.

Not all cases have such a happy ending however and the next case study illustrates this, where despite great efforts and good organisation the end result is not what is expected.

Case Study Two

Presentation

Mr Y, a 75-year-old man with evidence of arterio-sclerotic dementia, is brought to the attention of the psychiatrist by a family doctor who is concerned that the stress of looking after this man is making his wife depressed and physically unwell. The couple live by themselves and have some family but they are living some 350 miles away and cannot help in the current situation. Mr Y has been recently accused of being noisy and disruptive by his immediate neighbours whom he believes on occasions are trying to run his life.

Current Problems

The Patient. Mr Y is going through episodes of lucidity but these are becoming less frequent. He is continent but ignores his personal hygiene to the extent that he smells offensive. His sleep pattern is disturbed and he eats little nourishing food.

The Patient's Wife. Mrs Y, herself somewhat frail, is finding it increasingly hard to cope with her husband. She has no control over him and he will not co-operate with her on such matters as personal hygiene, mealtimes and sleep.

The Team

The care team is presented with a man who is in danger of being rejected by the community support that he has. This will lead inevitably to his admission to hospital for which he is not yet ready. Help is needed to organise assistance for Mrs Y and to provide a community back-up service which will allow Mr Y a longer life in the community.

The Decision

The team decide to admit Mr Y for seven days to a psychogeriatric assessment centre in order that he can be assessed fully and that Mrs Y can have seven days of much-needed rest. Mr Y agrees to admission and goes to the local psychogeriatric centre for short-term stay and assessment. Mrs Y agrees to have her home assessed and a record made of her timetable of daily events.

The Problems

There are three basic problem areas:

(1) Mr Y is markedly deteriorating and has little or no way of coping with his daily life. He must be directed to carry out most of his activities of daily living.
(2) Mrs Y has a daily timetable which still expects Mr Y to contribute actively within it in such areas as decision-making and planning. She cannot easily reconcile herself to the fact that he can no longer contribute in these areas.
(3) Mr Y is testing the limits of the tolerance of the neighbourhood by being mildly abusive towards them and accusing them of things which they have not done.

The Plan

This also has three aspects:

(1) When Mr Y is discharged from the psychogeriatric assessment ward he will be visited daily by a community nurse who will prepare him in order that he can be ready to go to the local day hospital five mornings a week.
(2) Mrs Y is given telephone numbers in order that she can contact the team personnel day or night if she needs advice or assistance.
(3) Mrs Y is to reorganise her daily timetable so that it allows her to make the decisions and organise the day's events around her coping ability.

There will be a team review in three weeks' time

The Proceedings

Mr Y was visited daily by the community nurse and was managing (with much ill will) to attend the local day hospital.

Mrs Y has now reorganised her lifestyle to cope with Mr Y's disabilities. She has used the telephone facility only twice and on each occasion managed the particular situation after a telephone conversation with one of the team.

Three Week Evaluation

The team decides that it is in order to change the programme so that the community nurse is not so heavily committed by the daily visiting. The home nursing service has agreed to share the load with the community psychiatric nurse visiting on alternate days for one week; it will then eventually take over all together. In detail, it is decided that:

(1) The community psychiatric nurse will phase out the daily visits over the next three weeks.
(2) Mr Y is to continue visiting the day hospital for the next four weeks.
(3) Mrs Y is to maintain her contact by telephone if needed.

Evaluation is to be made again in four weeks' time.

Proceedings

On the next day when the community psychiatric nurse visited, Mr Y had jumped from his bedroom window and killed himself five minutes before the nurse arrived.

Comments

The best-laid plans do not always cater for the unexpected and however many contingency plans are prepared there is no way to allow for events such as this.

We raised four major issues when considering programme planning, but this case study perhaps produces a fifth. However valiant the efforts, not all cases can be happily resolved. A well-planned programme of itself does not provide a new set of convenient solutions. It is however providing a route to follow and a foundation on which to build care delivery so that it may be more effectively and efficiently given.

Evaluation

The final piece of the jigsaw in care delivery is programme evaluation. There are a number of facets to patient outcome, some more important than others but all worthy of at least passing consideration. Evaluation is a measure of worth, an indicator of success and a pointer to future activity. Unfortunately, evaluation often receives little more than a token acknowledgement from many care-givers and may be tacked on to the end of a programme as an afterthought. It is the authors' belief that evaluation deserves more thought than this and should feature more prominently in mental health care. What follows is an overview of the field of evaluation and an examination of some selected aspects in greater detail.

The Patient's View

Who better than the recipients of a treatment can say how effective it has been? They alone have experienced the treatment event; their comments must therefore have some validity. There is no greater temptation than to ignore the comments of patients, for after all they are the unfortunate sufferers of a mental disorder which must make their judgement suspect! Any untoward comments about a programme can therefore be safely shrugged off as distorted and valueless. This is not necessarily true. Research work has in fact been undertaken in two areas: informal comments as to a programme's effectiveness have been collected (see Gurin *et al.*, 1960) and standardised questionnaires reinforced by interview have also been used (see Mental Handicap Studies Research Report, 1980).

Clinical Evaluation

A clinical evaluation is that type of evaluation which is carried out by those using some sort of professional judgement, for example rating scales of behaviour and measurements of change in the patient's state. Nurses, doctors, social workers and psychologists all have various approaches to dealing with this topic and this will be dealt with in greater detail further on.

Cost/Benefit and Effectiveness Techniques

This approach to evaluation has to be dealt with at a slightly different level than the two preceding approaches. Is the effort or the return worth the money invested or are there cheaper methods available which will have a greater or more positive effect than those being used? The current enthusiasm for evidence of a good return for money invested makes this an increasingly important area for those operating in the community with the mentally disordered. Is community care more beneficial than hospital care and how economically viable is it to expect the community to care for its own? At what point in time is it most beneficial to hand over responsibility of care to a family or back to the individual? (See Dawe, 1980 and Levin *et al.*, 1977.)

Mental Health Programme Effectiveness

This is to some extent a combination of areas listed so far. The current enthusiasm for discharge into the community of large numbers of ex-hospital residents and the treatment of greater numbers of people actually being cared for in the community pose a number of questions:

(1) Are appropriate resources being channelled into the community to cater for the extra demand?
(2) Can the community cope with this new approach and if not how can it be helped?
(3) Is all this good for the patient?
(4) Is all this good for the community?

For the purposes of this book we will concentrate upon clinical evaluation and patient's self-evaluation and to this end these two areas will be looked at in greater detail.

Evaluation in fact depends very heavily upon initial assessment and a division of the two is artificial. Evaluation is in essence another assessment taken at a period after a treatment programme has been in action for some time. If you cannot identify the original state which existed when treatment started, it then becomes impossible to say how much progress you have made and what the next step should be.

What Do We Need to Evaluate?

Objective Data

We need to consider the question: what can this person do now that he could not do before the start of the programme? The answer obviously depends upon the deficits that the person had to start with. An example can be drawn from a person who is withdrawn, mute and cannot hold conversations. After a period of relationship formation and social skills training, tests can be carried out to ascertain how far the person has progressed; and some scale can then be given to his performance (see Figure 6.2).

Figure 6.2: Progress of Withdrawn, Mute Client

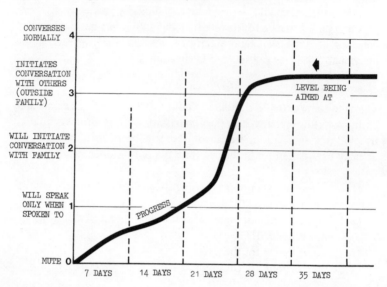

The level being aimed at may be level 3 where the man can initiate conversation with other people. Once this level is reached the programme can stop, for the level may be the optimum for this person. To attempt going beyond this point is perhaps asking the impossible and wasting resources.

A second example may be drawn from a person who has little or no domestic ability (see Figure 6.3). If this person is to live with some sort of self-sufficiency, he or she must learn these skills in order to survive. Once again the optimum performance may be at level 3 and there is no need to progress beyond this point. To master basic cooking skills can be enough to survive in the community and cordon bleu rosettes are not a prerequisite for self-sufficiency.

These task-defined evaluations are easy enough to measure given a well-defined baseline from which to start. The procedure becomes a little more complex where there are a multiple of such areas to assess. Complex problems are the most common, and to represent these accurately for evaluation will present some difficulty.

Efforts have been made to provide an all-embracing assessment which allows for a periodic evaluation (Markson and Allen, 1976) over given periods of time. Not only do these attempt to evaluate a number of different areas, but they also provide a scoring system which when completed gives the care-giver a 'word picture' according to the score obtained. The top score, 91-100, indicates: 'No symptoms, superior functioning in a wide range of activities, life's problems never seem to get out of hand, is sought out by others because of his warmth and integrity'. The bottom score of 1-10 indicates: 'Needs constant supervision for several days to prevent hurting self or others, or makes no attempt at personal hygiene'. This is an interesting and under-researched area which warrants further investigation.

Figure 6.3: Progress of Client Lacking Domestic Skills

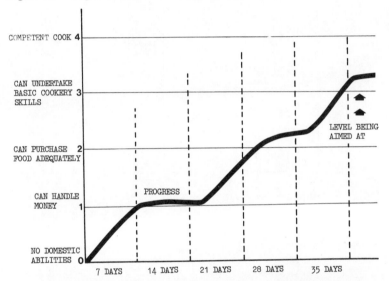

In that it is the authors' belief that there is no perfect formula yet developed for evaluations, what is the best way of developing a multi-problem evaluation system? The first rules must be: (1) keep it simple, (2) test it out and (3) observe the principles of questionnaire design (these will help the assessor over the pitfalls of badly worded or misleading areas for assessment). An outline approach is given in Figure 6.4 of potential areas and a possible scale.

Evaluation always appears to be overstating the obvious and therefore potential users may be put off by its 'insult' factor. The only argument to counter this is to try it first and criticise it second. Follow the steps outlined here and there will be every chance that you are setting out on the right foot:

114 *Programme Planning and Evaluation*

(1) Obtain an accurate baseline from initial assessments.
(2) Record data (preferably in a problem-orientated form) so that progression can be monitored.
(3) Evaluate regularly even if this is carried out informally.
(4) Evaluate each problem area and document the modified plan organised in the light of evaluations.
(5) Have a stated 'target, goal' system beyond which you will not or cannot go.

Figure 6.4: Outline of Multi-problem Evaluation System

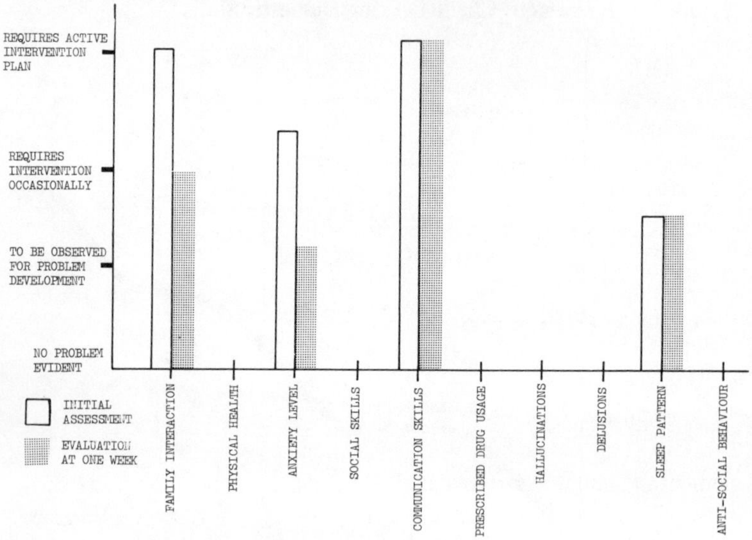

[Bar chart with y-axis categories: REQUIRES ACTIVE INTERVENTION PLAN; REQUIRES INTERVENTION OCCASIONALLY; TO BE OBSERVED FOR PROBLEM DEVELOPMENT; NO PROBLEM EVIDENT. Legend: INITIAL ASSESSMENT, EVALUATION AT ONE WEEK. X-axis categories: FAMILY INTERACTION, PHYSICAL HEALTH, ANXIETY LEVEL, SOCIAL SKILLS, COMMUNICATION SKILLS, PRESCRIBED DRUG USAGE, HALLUCINATIONS, DELUSIONS, SLEEP PATTERN, ANTI-SOCIAL BEHAVIOUR.]

Subjective Data

The patient's view of how he himself feels at a particular point in a programme of care is often a good guide as to the suitability of the pace and content of the programme. An example is drawn here from a patient who was undergoing domestic skills training and was asked to enter a shop and purchase potatoes. Minutes later she came out of the shop without the potatoes and reported to the trainer that there were none for sale. Going into the shop he pointed out several sacks of potatoes whereupon the patient exclaimed in dismay that she had not seen raw potatoes before as she had lived her whole life in institutions and had seen only cooked potatoes in a serving dish.

Here is a clear example of a programme going well but for one snag, the patient! Everyone has forgotten to involve her in her programme and assumptions are made about her level of knowledge.

Some rehabilitation programmes are very suspect. Ballroom dancing skills and basket weaving are often the prime concerns of many patients' day, neither of which will be of specific use for some cases when they return to the community.

Subjective self-evaluation covers the following areas:

(1) How happy are the patients with the programme?
(2) How well do they think they have done?
(3) Can they manage with the pace of the programme?
(4) Do they feel sufficiently involved?

Subjective data cast light on areas which are important but at the same time contentious. It may be that deficits are exposed in a programme and the outcome of this will rest upon the care-giver's ability to accept blame (where it is due) and to be flexible enough to change a programme approach. A case study can perhaps illustrate this best.

Case Study

Presentation

Mr W was a 63-year-old man who was initially referred to the psychiatrist by the court for (i) actions likely to cause offence and (ii) indecent exposure. Upon assessment Mr W was found to be progressively dementing, but at that particular time self-sufficient to the point of being able to live alone and cater for himself. Following his discharge from the psychiatric hospital, Mr W went to live with his daughter and her husband and their four children (twins aged six, one aged four and another aged eight). Mr W was re-referred as the family doctor was concerned that he might be arrested again, as he had been seen (informally) exposing himself to children in a local park.

Team Assessment

The care team assessed various aspects of the family and the following picture emerged. Mr W, who was currently tranquillised, was proving to be a problem at home as he was making vague sexual advances towards the young girls in the house. They had been instructed most precisely by their mother never to be on their own with him and to report to their mother if he made advances towards them. They were never left by the mother on their own in the house. The episodes were referred to as 'Grandad's games' and treated openly and with honesty by all involved. Mr W was never scolded but treated as ill and therefore in need of special attention. However the matter was *never* discussed with Mr W himself. The mother stated that her father's behaviour had been getting worse and he was now making advances in front of her, and went out much more often. He was also becoming a focus of torment from local boys who pursued him home and threw stones at him. There was a strong and loving bond between all members of the family including Mr W.

Problems

These were essentially that:
(1) Mr W was becoming more overt in his sexual advances to the children.
(2) Mr W was out on his own more often and in immediate danger of being arrested again (if observed or caught).
(3) The family, although coping magnificently, had limitations which could not be exceeded.
(4) The family did not want to break with Mr W and wished him to remain with them as long as possible.

The Plan

This involved three areas:

(1) Mr W's tranquillising medication to be increased and the family and a sexually-inhibitive drug regime to be commenced. The family and day hospital will administer the medication.
(2) Mr W is to attend day care, temporarily to keep him away from potential trouble areas.
(3) Mr W is to be drawn into the discussion and his problem behaviour pointed out. A record is to be kept by his daughter of his sexual behaviour in the home.

The plan is to be evaluated in four weeks' time.

The Proceedings

Drug therapies were initiated and maintained and Mr W, when interviewed by a social worker, apparently had little appreciation of his behaviour and became angry when pressed on the matter. Mr W attended the day centre regularly, thereby reducing to a minimum his

Programme Planning and Evaluation 117

opportunity for indecent exposure. His sexual activity continued at home but was reducing somewhat over the four weeks.

The Four Week Evaluation

A number of areas were evaluated to test the progress of the case and these are illustrated in Figures 6.5 and 6.6.

Figure 6.5: Multi-problem Evaluation of Progress of Mr W

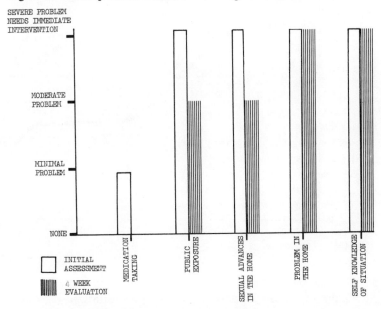

The current problems were seen to be:

(1) Although decreasing, Mr W's sexual advances in the home are still a problem.
(2) Mr W has little or no insight into his activity. Upon discussion he becomes very anxious and upset.
(3) The day hospital has relieved the situation at home considerably, but its facility is on limited offer only and a more permanent day arrangement must be found.

The revised plan involved:

(1) Continuing the current medication regime and monitoring of

sexual activities at home.
(2) Long-term day care facility to be found.
(3) Evaluation in a further four weeks and a self-rating evaluation to be given to the family at that time.

Figure 6.6: The Record of Mr W's Sexual Exposures in the Home

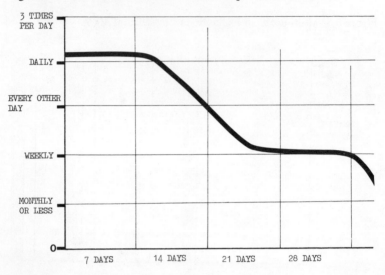

Further Proceedings

Mr W's behaviour continued to modify. The episodes of 'games' with the children decreased and none was reported in the final week before the next evaluation. No alternative day care was found for Mr W and this was compounded by the fact that his present day place was being pressurised by the authorities for people considered to be in greater need.

The Evaluation

The family members presented a self-rating scale devised by the team which examined their feelings about various areas:

(1) Management at home of Mr W.
(2) Effects on family life.
(3) Safety of the children.
(4) Capacity to supervise medication.
(5) How they might cope if Mr W came home permanently.

Figure 6.7: Team Evaluation of Progress of Mr W

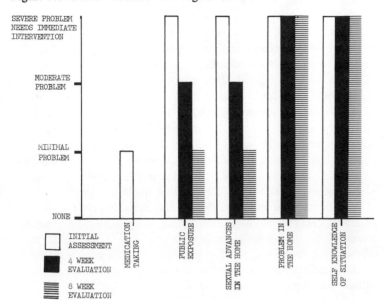

The team evaluation is shown in Figure 6.7. Thus the team still considered Mr W to be a problem in two main areas: (1) a management problem in the home, and (2) his lack of self-knowledge of the situation. This was not remotely supported by the family self-evaluation. They felt that they could cope most effectively with him as he now was, and there was enough strength in the family to support him without day care.

Therefore the next week Mr W was discharged to the care of his family (without day care). The community psychiatric nurse would visit each week for six weeks and then discharge Mr W if there were no problems.

Comments

There exists in this case an eventual division between the professional carers and the family. The assumption is that the family cannot yet cope with Mr W, but the family states through its self-evaluation that it can now do so. Without the use of this self-evaluation, the team might have made strenuous but needless efforts to place Mr W in day care and provide a longer care programme than it eventually did.

Getting Value For Money?

Economics and health services are not easy bed fellows. However, transposition of the economist's concepts and techniques to the health services has produced an interesting situation.

Health care is enormously expensive and getting more so as time goes on. New approaches to care are going to be carefully scrutinised by those who hold the access to funding. Community mental health care has two sides to it. First, exist the services which have always been to hand, the family doctor and the primary health care team. Secondly, however, new influences are afoot, which seek to place greater emphasis upon community care and draft into the community setting facilities which have otherwise only been available in the institutional setting.

To decide what is economically feasible and what is the right amount of care that can be delivered requires sophisticated approaches in order that both the economic and humanistic elements can be suitably satisfied. How far can a programme go? At what point is intervention too costly for the benefits it is providing. Three areas are briefly outlined here for the care-givers' consideration.

Cost/Benefit Analysis (CBA)

CBA seeks to determine the desirability of projects over a period of time. It takes account of the costs of mounting care programmes and values the relevant outcomes over a period of time. In this way the costs and benefits are compared to establish whether or not a care programme is worth mounting in the first place. Community care for the mentally disordered has been launched without any extensive consideration of this approach. The run-down of large hospitals which are disastrously expensive to run is an attractive proposition. Their replacement by locally-based community facilities has in many instances not been carried out, thus making community care an attractive proposition. Were the right tools available, a comprehensive CBA approach to this area would highlight that perhaps the community movement is not as beneficial as it appears from the surface, especially when one tries to cost-in the psychosocial burden on the family.

Cost Effectiveness Analysis (CEA)

The measurement and valuation of all costs and benefits is a difficult task in the health care system. CEA looks at the problem slightly differently. It requires the prior setting of goals and then tries to identify the way in which these goals can be met at the least cost, or in a way which the goals can best be achieved to the highest level for a given cost. This approach does not tell whether or not the care programme is worth mounting in the first place, but does identify the best or cheapest way of achieving its ends.

Programme Planning and Budgeting (PPB)

Programme planning and budgeting has general principles which can be widely applied to areas such as health and social services. Using the system, expenditure and work carried out are tied in with programmes which have measurable objectives. This allows a monitoring of progress and in the long term allows the development of the best and hopefully the cheapest ways of achieving programme objectives. The relevance of the preceding parts of this chapter can be seen as part of a system in which PPB might be implemented.

There is a general tendency in health care to avoid the planned approach to care and discount the importance of finance in care delivery, at least when there is a state-subsidised system. The heady days of the ever-open purse are over and there is no doubt that increasing pressure will be placed upon care-givers to recognise accountability in their everyday work. Planned programmes and evaluations are an integral part of this area; they not only supply a means of organising care but keep a check on effectiveness of care for the patient and the suppliers of the service.

References

Butterworth, C.A. (1981) 'Nurse Definition of Chronicity in Community Psychiatry' (Paper awaiting publication)
Dawe, A. (1980) 'To Be Or Not To Be', *CPNA Journal* (February), 10-12
Gurin, G., Verof, J. and Field, S. (1960) *Americans View their Mental Health* (Basic Books, New York)
Henderson, V. (1966) *The Nature of Nursing* (Macmillan, New York)
Levin, L.S., Katz, A.H. and Holst, E. (1977) *Self Care, Lay Initiatives in Health* (Croom Helm, London; Prodist, New York)
Markson, E.W. and Allen, D.F. (1976) *Trends in Mental Health Evaluation* (Lexington Books, Massachusetts)
Mental Handicap Studies Research Report (1980) Department of Mental Health, University of Bristol

Further Reading

Markson, E.W. and Allen, D.F. (1976) *Trends in Mental Health Evaluation* (Lexington Books, Massachusetts)

AUTHOR INDEX

Abel-Smith, B. 23, 31
Allen, D.F. 112, 121

Balint, M. 20, 21
Bandura, A. 44
Beishon, R.J. 54, 63
Borus, J.F. 37, 44
Bradshaw, J. 20, 21
Brown, G.W. 33, 44
Burke, J. 26, 31
Bursten, B. 40, 44
Butterworth, C.A. 37, 44, 49, 101, 121

Cambrill, E. 55, 63
Cameron, J. 26, 31
Camp, J. 23, 31
Caplan, G. 33, 35, 72, 73, 97
Carr, P.J. 37, 44
Cassell, E.J. 23, 31
Craddock, D. 27, 31

Davies, M. 52, 63
Davis, F. 14, 15, 21, 33, 44, 72, 75
Dawe, A. 111, 121
D'Espo, R. 40, 44
Douglas, M. 16, 21

Ferris, P. 22, 31

Gahan, K.A. 50, 63
Gellerman, S. 40, 45, 67, 71
Gleisner, J. 37, 45
Goffman, E. 40, 45
Gurin, G. 110, 121

Harris, T. 33, 44
Henderson, V. 99, 121
Hippocrates 24, 31

Illich, I. 23, 26, 31, 40, 45

Janis, I. 20, 21, 28, 32
Jobling, R. 21

Kane, R.L. 50, 32

Lee, L. 23, 32
Leigh, H. 34, 45

Levin, L.S. 33, 45, 111, 121
Lewis, I.M. 13, 16, 21
Lewis, J.M. 52, 63
Ley, P. 25, 32
Lindmann, E. 33, 45
Lippman, W. 17, 21
London, P. 65, 97
Lyall, W.A.L. 37, 45

MacLean, U. 15, 21
McWhinney, I.R. 35, 45
Marks, I. 66, 97
Markson, E.W. 112, 121
Marris, B. 72, 97
Mechanic, D. 34, 45
Miller, J. 13, 21

Osmond, H. 83, 97

Parry, J. 22, 32
Parry, N. 22, 32
Peters, G. 54, 63
Peterson, D.R. 65, 97
Pollack, K. 23, 32

Reiser, M.R. 34, 45
Richardson, C. 18, 21
Richman, J. 14, 21
Rope, J.A. 79, 91, 97
Rosenhan, D.L. 18, 21
Roth, J. 15, 21
Ryback, R.S. 50, 63

Scheff, T.J. 30, 32
Shaw, G.B. 23, 32
Shaw, R. 78, 97
Siegler, M. 83, 97
Skidmore, D. 14, 19, 20, 21, 25-7, 30, 32, 42, 45, 56, 63, 98
Solzhenitsyn, A. 77, 98
Spelman, M.S. 25, 32
Stockwell, F. 26, 32
Stoker, M.J. 14, 21, 30, 32, 42, 44, 45, 56, 63, 65, 69, 78, 82, 98

Underwood, E.A. 23, 32

Waddington, I. 27, 32
Weed, L.L. 50, 63

Wightman, W.P.D. 23, 32
Wolley, F.R. 50, 63

Zola, I. 15, 21

SUBJECT INDEX

abuse
   child 93-4
   wife 93
agoraphobia 66, 69, 83
alcoholism 95
Apothecaries 22, 26
approach laws
   of treatment 71
   in evaluations 113
assessment
   and treatment 67
   as seen by incrementalists 49
   as seen by universalists 50
   environmental 56
   functional 56
   general/clinical 55
   of family 59
   social 56

'bandwaggon effect' of client treatment 65
Barber Surgeons 22
biofeedback 92

care giving 22
   and history 22-5
   and humanism 23
   in hospital 22
case studies
   (Mr W) using a planned approach 115-19
   (Mr Y) using aims and objectives 107-9
   (Mrs Z) using aims and objectives 104-7
client 26-9, 64-75, 82, 85
   differences between 28-9
   expectations 28
   relationships 28-30, 43, 67
   status 69
   sick role 75
   taking up services 34
community care 26, 27, 30, 31
   and history 26
consultation habits 34
cost effectiveness 120
   and analysis 121
   and benefit 120
crisis 33, 42, 44, 72, 77

development of 75, 76
family in 74
types of 73

decision making 40, 44, 67
   in planned programmes 101-3
deviance 16-18, 40
   and predjudice 17
   as a process 16, 17
   image of 16
   road to 18
diagnosis 24, 66
   as a topographic function 55

evaluation
   and complex problems 112
   and PPB 121
   clinical 110
   guidance towards 115
   using objective data 111
   using subjetive data 114

family 38-44, 59, 68, 69, 72, 73
   assessment 59
   crisis 74
   roles 38
   security 39
   symbols 38
   therapy 40, 42-4, 75, 78, 91

GP (family doctor) 26, 27
   and storekeeping 27
gradual exposure 67, 83, 87-90, 93

Health Status index 33-4
hierarchy 87
hospital
   isolation 24
   specialism 23
   teaching 23
   voluntary 23
hospital care 22, 23, 24
   as a closed system 54
   as an open system 54

implosion 64, 83, 90
information giving 25, 26, 95
institutionalism 40, 75

Subject Index

labelling 14, 29, 39, 41, 67, 74, 92
    and prejudice 17
    and stigma 18
    as a symbol 15
lay network 25, 26
lay referral 18
learned helplessness 65, 75
levels of involvement 99
    phased levels 99-100
    with patients 99

medical arena 18-20
modelling 87
Murphy's law 42-3, 89

Ostler 64

patient career 15, 18-20, 26, 27, 40, 65
    expectations of 26, 28
    in hospital 19, 23, 25
    media and 26
    status of 27
phobia 64, 69
physicians 22
planned programmes
    and time scales 101
    goal setting 101
    involving patients 100
    use of aims 101-2
    use of objectives 102-3
polio 14
preventative medicine 24
problem orientated approaches (POR) 50-1
    and records 50
psychiatry
    and stigma 30
    differences in setting 31
    families and 39
    stigma 30
    use of media 30, 39
psychotic 91

relaxation 83, 84
    method of 84-6
rite of passage 27
ritual 13, 24, 26

self care 33
service provision 35
    primary care 35, 36
    secondary care 35, 36
    tertiary care 35-7

sexual dysfunction 92
sickness
    and family doctor 19
    as a symbol 15, 20
    behaviour in 14, 15
    care giving 22, 25
    information and 20, 65
    meaning of 13
    position aspect of 13
    school avoidance in 14
    specialist and 19
spider phobic 87
symbol 13, 22
systems theory
    and goal identification 52
    closed 54
    dynamic 54
    environmental factors in 52
    uncertainty of 52

timetables 64, 73, 76
treatment
    and education 92-4, 97
    approach law 71
    assessment of 67
    client centered 72
    commitment towards 70-1
    defining needs for 68
    honesty in 65, 70
    information and 68
    laws of 64, 66, 97
    management of 65
    responsibility for 65, 68, 72, 77, 82, 95, 98
Tuke 91

workhouse 23